MIRACLE STEM CELL HEART REPAIR

For Heart Attack, Heart Failure and Bypass Patients

By Christian Wilde

Abigon Press

BIBLIO DISTRIBUTION
(Division of National Book Network)

ISBN: 1-59975-054-6
ISBN (13) 978-1-59975-054-5

Library of Congress Control Number: 2006933014

PRINTED IN THE UNITED STATES OF AMERICA
First printing August, 2006
1 2 5 7 9 10 8 6 4 2

Edited By: Michael Frisoli, Ph.D., ENG. USC
Cover Design: Peri Poloni-Gabriel, Knockout Design
Illustrator: Jeeyoung
Book Design: Jack Hillman, Hillman Design Group

Preface

To Heart Disease Patients everywhere, your situation has not gone unnoticed and medical science has not forgotten that you and millions like you are hoping and praying for a miracle. Researchers, physicians, scientists, cardiologists, administrators and technologists from institutions all over the world have dedicated their lives to prolonging yours. Working tirelessly in an effort to mediate against this number one killer. Here then for your approval is their progress and their report card.

Christian Wilde

TABLE OF CONTENTS

Not enough angioplasties being done in a timely manner

A high risk interventional practice
Angiography
Progress in slowing heart disease
Left main surgery or left main angioplasty?
Getting to the meat of the meeting
Designer "off the shelf" cells

What is different about mesenchymal Cells?
The big picture
When is a stem cell a stem cell?
Your Magnificent Heart
Cardiac arrest/sudden death
Avoiding the heart lung machine

When science and religion coexist

Stem cells for diabetes
Stem cells for the eyes
Stem cells for macular degeneration
Stem cells for lungs
Stem cells for neurodegenerative disease
Stem cells for cancer
Stem cells for kidney disease
Stem cells for spinal injury
Stem cells for sickle cell

In Merck's own words

Heart failure improvement with Coenzyme Q10
Ejection fraction improvement in 84% of the study participants
Does Coenzyme Q10 improve survival rates?
Natural adjuvants for treatment of congestive heart failure
Canada convinced, orders warnings
Statin depleting effect on obiquinone, Coenzyme Q10

The annual cost to the health care system
Will the answer for angina come from stem cells?
What is the future for angina patients?
Reporting early study results
Stable angina or unstable angina?

Heart failure and Ace Inhibitors
Other ways Ace Inhibitors help extend life
A valuable ally for diabetic patients

The government statin side effect study
A non-inflammatory form of myopathy
Greater risk with longer statin use
Statin side effects are dose related, some patients may never
    recover
A two edged sword
Lessons from another dose related case
Natural alternatives for patients who cannot tolerate statins?
Cause and effect with taking drugs
Statins lower inflammation
Cholesterol too low?

Low cholesterol and greater risk of hemmoragic stroke

Understanding the kinds of strokes
Hemmoragic stroke
Ischemic stroke
TIA (transient ischemic attack)
Embolic stroke
Thrombatic stroke
Aspirin (ASA) and stroke
Low cholesterol linked to hostile, aggressive, violent behavior, depression
Low cholesterol and violent behavior, is it all in the head?
Statin and fibrate drugs together

ILLUSTRATIONS

Fig.1 Spinal injury repair. Courtesy Dr. Carlos Lima. Page 31

Fig. 2 Dark area denotes advanced plaque in an older mouse artery before VPC treatment. Page 48

Fig. 3 Note: Plaque is almost totally dissolved after treatment with VPC cells from a young healthy mouse. Page 49

Fig. 4 Skeletal muscle fiber. Page 59

Figs. 5 & 6 Duane's before and after 3-dimensional Noga Mapping scans show amazing and conclusive heart repair. See color images Figs. 8 and 9. Page 77

Fig. 7 Adjusting a predetermined catheter needle length Page 107

Color Illustrations

Fig. 8 Spinal injury repair. Page 145

Fig. 9 Dr. Cohen PET before and after results. Page 145

Fig. 10 The red area shows destroyed heart muscle from previous heart attack—the green denotes healthy tissue. The 3 black spots indicate where Duane's own stem cells were injected into his damaged heart. Page 146

Fig. 11 At 3 month follow-up using 3-dimensional Noga Mapping, the previous dead heart muscle (red) is shown replaced with viable healthy (green) heart tissue. Images appear by special permission. Before and after scanning performed with Cordis Noga Mapping. Page 147

Fig. 12 Dark area denotes advanced plaque in an older mouse artery before VPC treatment. Page 148

DISCLAIMER

Nothing you will be presented in this book is offered to replace or supercede your doctor's advice or treatment plan for you. The information is meant to be a reference source and an educational tool to prepare you for discussions with your physician. If you have been diagnosed with heart disease or have previously experienced a heart attack or stroke and if you would like to minimize additional risk, your doctor may find the information from highly respected researchers and physicians helpful. Medical information is updated continually and what one may read represented and accepted today may be challenged in the near future. All any author or researcher can reasonably do is to present the information from reliable sources as it appears in the literature. It is not the intent of the publisher to provide all of the information available on any given subject, you are encouraged to seek additional information. The author and publisher shall have neither liability or assumed responsibility for any alleged or actual damage caused by any information provided in this book in regard to any entity or individual. Certain applicable information from book one has been updated and included.

CHAPTER 1

The
Possible Impossible
Dream

*I*t seems like just yesterday that Microsoft's Bill Gates announced a new phenomenon he called "The Information Highway." Suddenly, as if overnight the internet was born and we all began acquiring a new vocabulary, a new language which includes words like download, modem, email, software, hard drives and on and on. The internet, whether we saw it as an intrusion or not, became an everyday part of our lives.

Many years ago a movie called *Jurassic Park* sent our youngsters running to the libraries and scanning the Internet to learn more about dinosaurs and the genetic scientific link to their past. In 2004, a tsunami transfixed our attention on television radio and newspaper reports. We were eager to educate ourselves to a better understanding of the scientific language that would help explain seismic changes, tectonic plates, gigatons and how transferred energy on an ocean floor could send water, at almost 600 miles an hour to an unsuspecting shoreline, hundreds of miles away. Now again another technology and science is upon us bringing yet another new language, challenging us once again to confront the future. This breakthrough is the exciting, absolutely amazing emerging science of heart stem cell research and application.

The author's task, then, is to help explain this science in everyday language and explore its promise. To do that, we will all need to hear from the recognized world authorities who are in the forefront leading the race. Several have generously contributed information to the book you are about to read: Joshua Hare, M.D., Director, Heart Failure and Cardiac Transplantation/Director, Cardiovascular Institute for Cell Engineering, Johns Hopkins University—Warren Sherman, M.D, FACC, FSCAI, Director, Cardiac Cell Based Endovascular Therapies, Columbia University, New York City—Timothy Henry, M.D., FACC, Minnesota Heart Institute Foundation, Minneapolis, Minnesota—Nabil Dib, M.D., MSc, FACC, Chief of Cardiovascular Research, Arizona Heart Institute, Phoenix, Arizona—Doris Taylor, Ph.D., Bakken Professor & Director, Center for Cardiovascular Repair, University of Minnesota—Amit Patel, M.D., MS, Director, Center Cardiac Cell Therapy, UPMC Medical Center, Director of Stem Cell Therapy, Pittsburgh Pennsylvania—Douglas Losordo, M.D., Chief Cardiovascular Research, St. Elizabeth Medical Center, Tufts University School of Medicine—Rajendra Makkar, M.D., Co-Director Catherization Laboratory and Co-Director, Cardiovascular Research, Cedars Sinai Medical Center, Los

Angeles, California. As you will become aware, there have already been more than 2,000 documented successful heart stem cell implantations in patients using their own stem cells. The word that continually is applied in explanation of the results is MIRACULOUS. We will share several of the patient's personal stories who have already successfully undergone a procedure enabling them to live fully functional lives once again. As with any breakthrough, what will be obviously missing from the current evaluations will be the very long-term results. Those of you and your supportive families who have been on this cardiovascular journey with you will surely relate and rejoice in hearing first-hand accounts from patients. These are fortunate individuals whose medical situation in a matter of weeks or a few short months transitioned from near death to triumph. Metaphorically speaking, if it can be said the scientist practices the art of medicine—he or she may be considered the artist, technology the canvas, and the patients you are about to meet, the finished painting. They share their stories in a desire to bring you hope.

During the five years I devoted to the previous research and writing of the *Hidden Causes of Heart Attack and Stroke,* the emphasis was on identifying and intervening against the hidden factors that lead to and complicate the long-term developing process of heart disease. The mandate was not only to identify the causes but to also provide solutions and strategies from the research community involving integrated medicine (a combination of pharmaceutical and natural medicine). Heart disease is now considered to be 90% preventable. However, as vital as the preventive information presented in the book was in helping to avert a crisis or need for major intervention, questions still remained.

These are questions articulating concerns affecting those particular patients whose disease already was, or is now, becoming far advanced. Patients who received the preventive information very late in the disease process and may already have found themselves among the epidemic 5M congestive heart failure patients in America. Perhaps a patient who has previously experienced one or more myocardial infarctions (heart attacks) and lives each day with the conscious or subconscious realization that his/her magnificent heart that has served them so well—faithfully pumping 100,000 times a day, 36,400,000 times in a given year and producing enough blood in a lifetime to fill 3 ½ giant oil tankers–is now losing its ability to function! A heart that is failing as a result of inflicted damage from previous heart attacks or uncontrolled chronic high blood pressure or possibly advanced atherosclerosis. What hope is there for the patient who has heard the final decree from their physician, "We have done all we medically know how to do in your care." Are you one of these patients? Does someone you love or care about fall into one of these unenviable categories and is in need of a miracle? A friend, father, mother, spouse, other relative, or possibly even yourself?

The Value of Life

No one has to tell the surviving victim of a heart attack that life is precious, frail and tentative. Regardless of how you valued or did not value it before the illness, it can no longer be taken for granted. As the Joni Mitchell song from the 70's, *Big Yellow Taxi* proclaimed, "Don't it always seem to go, you don't miss what you've got till it's gone." Even though a victim is on their way to recovery, they often suffer from severe anxiety and depression—learning that they may never be quite the same and they face a battle that has only begun.

Besides being an obvious physical attack there is also a spiritual component involved as one is confronted with their own mortality—as several of the patients whose stories you will read have mentioned. Their lives hung in the balance as they fought minute by minute to hold on. When people are asked to look back at their crises, they realize what a life altering experience a heart attack is, particularly, when they comprehend the odds that were stacked against their very survival. The incalculable odds, that if someone hadn't summoned the paramedics at the right exact moment, if the paramedics had arrived late by overshooting the address a few blocks, or mistakenly ending up at South Main Street instead of North Main, and if a friend or family member hadn't been there in the meantime to intervene with CPR, they quite simply would have been an added statistic in the county records that collectively record the more than 400,000 deaths by heart attack per year in America.

The numbers don't lie, they don't exaggerate. The national health organizations inform us that of these 400,000 deaths, 250,000 of the victims did not even survive the first hour after the onset of the attack. Physicians, while explaining the difficult and tenuous road ahead will soon be able to offer their patients very encouraging news. The use of one's own stem cells to repair the previously unrepairable heart!

As vitally important as the understanding of preventive heart healthcare is, a very sobering fact resounds, until now there has not been hope for regeneration of a heart damaged by a heart attack. The common understanding has been that what is done is done and scar tissue will always remain dead scar tissue. As well, there has not been a known remedy for congestive heart failure with its international enrollment of 22 million cases, 5 million in the US. We continue to add more than 450,000 new cases per year in this country. What has been needed, quite simply, are MIRACLES! That is the one-word description continually encountered when discussing stem cell heart therapy. Invariably, someone will exclaim, "That sounds almost unbelievable, why haven't we been told about this discovery?" Another popular reaction, "this sounds like a miracle."

Claiming the Future Today

The wheels of medicine have moved notoriously slow throughout medical history. The acceptance and application of new information is dictated by a combination of both medical and ethical reasoning. Consequently, the research community is generally 10-20 (or even more) years ahead of what will one day become applicable as common practice in hospitals and doctors' offices.

To illustrate the point, consider that Hypocrites used aspirin for various applications in its most native form of acetylsalicylic acid that he prepared from the bark of a willow tree 400 years before Christ! Ironically, it would take a very long time until aspirin's ability to minimize blood clotting among heart attack patients would be recognized. Actually it was 1968, 2,268 years after the Greek physician began using aspirin when the AHA recommended taking a 325 mgs tablet to mediate against platelet aggregation (clot formation) during a heart attack. Visionaries like Hypocrites and the many who brave the new frontiers of cardiovascular research today are not contained by the status quo but seek to develop and prove advanced modalities and technologies where others are content to justify their own lack of vision. The latter hold to a safe position with declarations like, "If it could have been done, somebody would have already done it!"

If you are like me you still marvel each time you observe

a giant jet airliner leaving the tarmac. Somewhere in the roar of the turbines a naysayer's voice from 1903 can still almost be heard, "If God had meant for man to fly, he would have given him wings." It has taken 51 years to gain FDA approval for one particular alternative bypass procedure we will be discussing called EECP®. Unfortunately, many who need life preserving or lifesaving information need it and need it now as they confront the reality that time may not always be a friend. There have been times (although rare) in the past, when the government agency, recognizing a group of patients with no other hope for survival, modifies the approval process through a compassionate provision allowing terminal patients the benefit of a relatively new therapy. After reading about many in congestive heart failure who are in the third or fourth stage of diagnosis one might wonder how heart stem cells for heart failure already proven successful in turning around such cases, can be withheld? What could possibly be the downside? What possible reason could there be in not permitting these patients and their doctors this last ray of hope?

Nonetheless, government dictates for patient safety, governed by the regulatory processes for patient safety in general, are vitally necessary to restrain over enthusiasm and to protect against mere speculation. Still, on occasion, even as stringent and thorough as the guidelines may be, there will be a breakdown in the process and a dangerous drug like Vioxx®, potentially linked to

140,000 non-fatal heart attacks and an actual 56,000 heart attack deaths—or a drug like the cholesterol lowering Baycol®, suspected to have killed 31 patients--will, regardless of all the examination and scrutiny, somehow gain approval. Incidentally, to put those 56,000 deaths by heart attack in perspective, the total losses of American lives during the entire Vietnam War added up to 55,000.

The good news for many patients is that the technological advancements for the detection and treatment of cardiovascular disease is moving forward at an amazing record-setting pace. Procedures that didn't seem even remotely possible as recently as five or ten years ago are right now being employed in the battle. Even though many of the stem cell procedures we will be discussing do not appear to be that far away from qualifying for final FDA approval, they are actually being performed successfully at this very time in the course of ongoing studies across the country. It is important for every heart patient and health provider to become aware of the possibilities and to be informed and ready to take advantage of what is coming available.

I believe you will embrace, as did I, these breakthroughs as being nothing short of revolutionary. Seeing is believing and hope is a free ride. Dr. Tim Henry, Director of Research at the Minneapolis Heart Institute estimates there are probably 1,000 successful cases of stem cell heart implantation in this country and another 1,000 or so overseas. The total numbers are increasing daily as more and more patients are entering the various trials. You will read several patients' stories that, to say the least, are convincing and inspiring. As one patient told me during an interview, "I could hardly walk to the bathroom without being winded and now four months after treatment, I walk two to four miles a day and don't even give my heart a second thought!"

How Many People Await This New Technology?

According to the American Heart Association database there are some 1,100,000 people who have had a heart attack in any given year, of that number approximately 400,000 survive. From a purely theoretical standpoint, if one were to extrapolate, multiplying collectively all the 400,000 per year heart attack survivors over the last 20 years—plus the 5M living with congestive heart failure today, the total number of people living with a damaged heart and needing a miracle in this country alone would stagger the imagination. Now add the 22 million who are suffering heart failure worldwide and all the surviving victims of heart attacks throughout the rest of the world and one begins to get a sense of how important any major breakthrough like stem cell heart repair really is. Remember heart disease is not just the number one killer in America but also the number one killer the world over.

CHAPTER 2

What is a Stem Cell?

• Every tissue in our body is constructed from stem cells and there are many kinds. These stem cells have the ability to replicate, to renew, to regenerate and to replace themselves as the body demands. As an example of our need for constant repair, even the simple act of exercise destroys or damages cells that will need to be replaced. As we age, our bodies become less efficient in producing cells to meet the demand and our production falls behind the curve. Aging begins to take its toll. The deficit expresses itself in loss of brain cells, muscle mass and skin tone; the unwelcome formation of wrinkles; and the breakdown of vital organ tissue and organ function within the body. Unfortunately, degenerative and immune diseases can now more easily gain a foothold and begin their destructive process. The very process of aging, as well as the process controlling disease, is the result of a breakdown in cellular health. Cell types are identified by their strength, giving scientists an idea of their potential ability to heal. Following are a few of the cell types. I promise this discussion of cell types will be brief and the remainder of the book far less technical. Let's do a little homework to prepare us for the discussion. You will not be graded or even asked to take a test and that too is a promise!

- Totipotent stem cells are produced from the fusion of an egg and sperm cell. Cells produced by the first few divisions of the fertilized egg cell are also totipotent. These cells can grow into any type of cell without exception.

- Embryonic stem cells: Within their broad capacity lies a unique scientific challenge, how to differentiate (specialize) the cells to meet the requirements of a specific targeted therapy. As well, there are challenging clinical issues aside from any moral or ethical discussions that must be reconciled before ESC cells can successfully provide human benefit: a) finding a way to ameliorate an acknowledged propensity to develop tumors as has been the case to date in many animal studies, b) rejection, as they are derived from a foreign source and c) controlling (as has been reported) cell migration to the brain from the actual site of transplantation.

- Pluripotent stem cells are the descendants of totipotent stem cells and can grow into any cell type in the body but cannot actually produce a human being.

- Multipotent stem cells can produce only cells of a closely related family of cells as example blood cells: red blood cells, white blood cells and platelets.

- Unipotent cells can produce only one cell type, but have the property of self-renewal which distinguishes them from non-stem cells.

Where do Stem Cells Stem From?

Stem cells are also categorized according to their source, adult, embryonic or cord blood stem cells.

- Stem cells used in heart repair are adult stem cells and present no possibility for rejection, no moral implication regarding their harvesting and are proving to be very effective in treating many other diseases in addition to heart disease. They do not produce tumors and have the ability to survive for long periods of time and to prevail under hostile environmental conditions.

- Embryonic stem cells are cultured cells obtained from the undifferentiated inner mass cells of an early stage human embryo (sometimes called a blastocyst). The controversy lies in the fact that in order to start a stem cell line or lineage, it requires the destruction of a human embryo and/or therapeutic cloning which some believe may lead to reproductive cloning and could result in the objectification of a potential human being. In an attempt to overcome these moral, political and ethical hurdles, medical researchers have been experimenting with alternative techniques of producing embryonic stem cells, which do not involve cloning and/or the destruction of a human embryo.

• Cord blood stem cells are derived from the very rich blood source of the placenta and umbilical cord after birth. Umbilical cord blood banks for storage of a child's umbilical cord are becoming very popular.

The Cell Race

Any good horse race handicapper would advise one to study the horses carefully and to look at all their attributes, strengths and weaknesses before picking a winner, reminding us to remain open, acknowledging it is difficult, once committed, to change horses in mid-race.

The Nation's Introduction to Stem Cells

Most of us, relatively speaking were probably totally unaware of this medical phenomena called stem cell therapy until actor-activist, patient, Christopher Reeve brought it front and center—drawing us into his very personal battle with a paralytic condition of quadriplegia resulting from an equestrian accident several years earlier. Undoubtedly his celebrity brought attention from his fan base and from a compassionate public at large. His appearances before Congress requesting more funding for embryonic research brought further national attention. Although his physical malady would one day in the near future require stem cell implantation in his spine to repair spinal cord injury, the only source of those stem cells according to what was presented would be from embryonic cells. Any other form of stem cell was not introduced or included in the discussion. The world was talking about stem cells and that was a good thing.

Stem cells for fighting certain diseases like Parkinson's, MS, liver and diseases of the kidneys, eyes, brains and on and on. However, the message sent to the public through the advocacy seemed to say, it is all or nothing. Either using human embryos or not using them and seemingly condemned to remain in the dark ages of medicine. What was somehow unfortunately lost in this discussion was the hard work, benefits and progress researchers have been documenting using other forms of stem cells since the 1960's. In a scientific sense, the information dispensed to the public could have been more representative, complete and balanced, especially since human lives hang in the balance.

All of us listening to the beloved actor's declaration that he would one day walk again believed and hoped with him. It was a world in love with Superman wishing him total recovery by whatever form of technology it would take. With an eye truly on the prize it wouldn't matter where the cure would finally come from. Truth be known, had his accident occurred in the past two or three years and had he not met his untimely death from pneumonia he might well be walking or beginning to walk today. Christopher's miracle however, may not necessarily have come from embryonic stem cells as initially believed, but from his own stem cells. Quadriplegia is caused when the injury is in the cervical (neck) area of the spine. When the injury is sustained in the cervical region, the person may lose mobility in the arms as well as the legs. Paraplegia affecting the legs can be the result of an injury to the lower back. Spinal injury patients may find a ray of hope in hearing the following examples of patients who are walking after doctors treated their condition with adult cells from their own bodies.

Laura Dominguez in 1991 was left a quadriplegic, as was Christopher, as a result of an accident. She later benefited from an adult stem cell procedure using her own cells. The surgery was performed at Egaz Moniz Hospital, in Lisbon Portugal by Dr. Carlos Lima. Three years ago he had already performed cell transplant surgery on six individuals. Three were quadriplegics and four paraplegics. Six of the seven had what were classified as complete injuries. Dr. Lima's successful surgeries are now approaching thirty.

Stem Cells for Spinal Injury

- The doctor and his team had harvested olfactory sinus stem cells from Laura's nose transplanting them into the damaged areas of her spine. At last report Laura was walking, although with the help of braces. According to a report by Bradley Hughes Jr, "Laura became the 10th patient to benefit from this surgery and the second American. After a post-surgical MRI had been done, physicians informed her that her spinal cord had begun healing and that 70 percent of the lesion had recovered into normal spinal tissue." According to the Hughes report, "Within six months Laura had acquired sensation down to the abdominal region. By 2004 she had gained upper body agility and the ability to stand for extended periods of time although for now with the aid of a walker. In addition, she reported improved motor skills, including the ability to stand on her toes, contracting her quadriceps and hamstring muscles. She also announced that she had walked more than 1,400 feet with the use of braces. Laura, inspired by the results, hopes to walk

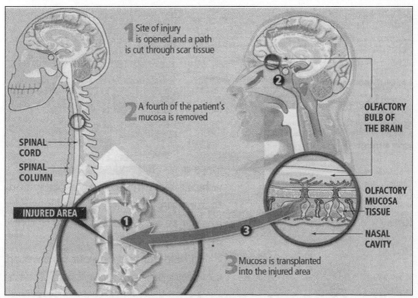

Fig.10 Spinal injury repair. Courtesy Dr. Carlos Lima.

unassisted by the time she turns 21." I caught up with Dr. Lima in Italy and asked a question that I am sure he had been asked many times. If Christopher Reeve had not met his untimely death from pneumonia, could his have possibly been a case that might have benefited from the olfactory cell transplant? Dr. Lima responded by sharing with me a recent case of a young man whose injury was very similar to the actor's but happened just two years ago. The young man from Chicago had been shot in the high cervical area of his spine. After giving the boy olfactory stem cell treatment, said Lima, "he is already able to remain off the ventilator 12 hours a day."

• In still another remarkable case reported in the *Korean Times*, researchers at Chosun University in Souel, South Korea, documented an outcome in which a woman who had not been able to stand for the previous 19 years began to walk, following umbilical cord stem cell implantation. According to the report, a team of Korean researchers claimed they had performed a miracle by enabling a patient to walk with stem cell therapy, using multipotent umbilical cord cells. Three weeks following the procedure the patient began walking!

These are just two examples of progress being made using adult stem cells for spinal injury. The Korean miracle utilized a technology involving stem cells from umbilical cord blood and Laura Domingues' miracle came from stem cells from her own nose tissue. None of these miracles came from embryonic therapy. Why haven't we all heard more about these cases and so many more similar successes? Why aren't they front-page news?

What is perhaps most amazing of all and of concern to you and I today is the marvelous progress being made in damaged heart restoration. While stem cells, thankfully, are currently being studied for treatment of all manner of disease including Lou Gherig's, Alzheimer's, MS, muscular dystrophy, diabetes, Parkinson's and even neuromuscular disease, it is the diseases of the human heart that is the focus of this book. Wouldn't you agree that defeating the number one killer of people worldwide would be enough of a challenge for any type of stem cell? It would appear, according to the clinical evidence you are about to read, that the solution to heart damage just happens to lie in the area of adult stem cell repair.

According to the director of the National Genome Research Institute, Donald Orlic, as told to NBC news, "We are currently finding that these adult stem cells can function as well, perhaps even better than embryonic stem cells." Catherine M. Verfaillie, Ph.D., researcher and director of the University of Minnesota Stem Cell Institute, made her announcement, "a certain new type of stem cell can do anything an embryonic cell can do and perhaps even more." The University of Texas Medical School is scheduled to begin a first study to treat traumatic brain injury in children utilizing their own stem cells.

Adult Cells for Brain and Muscle Disorders?

On February 19, 2003, The *Journal of the American Medical Association* (JAMA) reporting on research from Johns Hopkins Medical School presented the information that donor stem cells for the first time crossed the blood brain barrier and became neurons in a recipient's brain. This is an important finding because neurons are the most highly advanced functional cells in the body. They control all brain and muscle functions. "This is a recent revolutionary discovery about the potential to repair and regenerate the human brain." Dr. Eric Olson emphasized, "Our traditional views need to be re-evaluated." These (adult) stem cells do not pit science against religion and politics against ethics and in no way do they pose a moral or ethical dilemma. What we are about to discuss are stem cells extracted from a patient's own thigh muscle or derived from the patient's own bone marrow to rejuvenate the heart. We will explore these technologies and their exciting results to date. It isn't a matter of being adversarial in trying to prove something wrong with embryonic cells that is at issue here; rather it is recognizing and acknowledging what is right with adult stem cells.

One may only contemplate how the information would have been received in the national mindset had stem cells from one's own body been included as part of the country's introduction to cell therapy. Not only the public but also many of the medical community in general have not been made aware of the progress being made in other areas of stem cell research. As Doris Taylor, Director of the Center for Cardiovascular Repair at the University of Minnesota (with more than 20 years in this field says), "It is no more unethical to transplant one's own cells than it is to have a hair transplant." Joshua Hare, lead researcher of biochemical studies at JHU Johns Hopkins University has amply reminded us in regard to borrowing stem cells from third parties, "Stem cells from donors is after all not new at all. When you think about it, we have been using donor bone marrow for years in fighting diseases like leukemia and lymphoma." There are stem cells from umbilical cord blood and other blood sources being explored that have received very little media attention. Dr. Verfaillie presented her study findings during a BBC News interview; "Umbilical cord blood is a rich source of stem cells that may afford several potentially important advantages over embryonic or fetal stem cells." She went on to discuss the possibility of these cells even replacing diseased neurons in central nervous system disorders. Ihor Lemischka, Associate Professor of Molecular Biology at Princeton University, was also quoted on the BBC program as saying in support of Dr. Verfaillie's claims, "These adult marrow cells can differentiate into pretty much everything that an embryonic stem cell can differentiate (develop) into." German scientists recently announced in the journal *Nature* from Georg-August University of Goettingen Germany, "Testicular cells harvested from the testes of mice have proven to behave like embryonic stem cells. If the same holds true in humans it could provide another controversy-free source of versatile cells for use in treating disease." Testicular cells would actually precede embryonic cells in the chain of early development.

CHAPTER 3

Voodoo Science or *Major Breakthrough?*

S o, as a person who has suffered a heart attack or has been diagnosed with any of the prior complications associated with heart disease, you might have certain questions you would like answered. Questions such as:

- What exactly is this new science, how practical is it and how well is the medical profession embracing it?

- When will stem cell implementation become commonplace therapy and very importantly, what can you share with us to help us believe in its efficacy?

- What hope—backed by clinical evidence—can you instill for those of us who have already sustained damage from one or more heart attacks or have been told there are no more options?

- What hope can you share with us whose hearts are failing because of congestive heart failure?

• Where is the information to benefit the patient who is being advised to undergo a second or possibly a third open-heart surgery even though they are now more frail and much older than when they first had the initial surgery 10, 15 or 20 years earlier? Are there alternatives to surgery?

Quite simply, to date, there has not been a remedy for the heart damaged as a result of a previous heart attack or chronic high blood pressure—two conditions that can hasten permanent weakness of the left ventricle and lead to congestive heart failure. No, in spite of all the procedures and devices science has developed, not until now has there been a viable long term "fix." There has been little hope for the patient who has exhausted all opportunities for adequate grafts for additional bypass surgery or in general does not qualify. Dr. Timothy Henry, Director of Research at the Minneapolis Heart Institute, has been concerned about patients who fall into this category. You and I will hear from two of Dr. Henry's patients who are doing well after having non-invasive EECP® (enhanced external counterpulsation) treatments. Dr. Taylor also has a particular interest in the science of gene therapy's potential in unlocking remedy for patients whose options are limited.

Beginning of the Myoblast Stem Cell Phenomenon

After relating a story of a patient whose life had literally been given back to him using his own stem cells through skeletal myoblast cell transplant, Doris Taylor, Ph.D., pioneer and visionary of myoblast stem cell transplants for heart repair, answered my first question, "What does it feel like to see something you conceptualized and dreamed of bringing to fruition over 14 years ago now actually translating to the saving of human lives?" "Obviously," she replied, "as you would imagine, it means a great deal to me. When I hear patients' stories or receive patients' letters, I am humbled that I have been lucky enough to be a part of a growing solution for people who have experienced one, or in some cases several heart attacks."

Professor Taylor, who serves as Director of the Center for Cardiovascular Repair at the University of Minnesota and formerly on the cardiology faculty at Duke University Medical Center, reminds us of the enormity of the health problem that affects more than 22 million people worldwide. These patients are currently living under a diagnosis of heart failure. "For many of these people," Dr. Taylor explained, "there is the loss of ability to enjoy even the simplest pleasures, such as playing with grandchildren or engaging in normal, enjoyable daily activities. Many of the things that make a life worth living are just no longer an option for these heart failure patients. Our goal has been to try and improve their lives and provide a new, better or even best possible treatment. All the other options that are available – medications and devices like a pacemaker or an LVAD (left ventricular assist device)—are designed to make the remaining healthy part of the heart function better. This cell transplantation technology is the only treatment that is aimed at the underlying problem and begins to repair damage to the injured heart. This work we are doing is fun, it's exciting, and it is moving forward in a way that I think is going to give us some definitive answers in the next couple of years. Reminiscing, the doctor explained how 12-14 years earlier, "During the time we were trying to develop this concept, no one, but no one, believed it could be done. To keep myself and our team in a positive frame of mind and focused on the task at hand, I posted a favorite quote by Gandhi on my office door. 'First they ignore you, then they laugh at you, then they fight you, then you win.' We are closer to winning and more importantly so are patients. What a privilege to make a difference in people's lives, particularly when it is an extension of our initial notion and premise, which was to try to make a positive difference, in helping somehow, to change the world."

Dr. Taylor shares this concept and hope with her colleagues in many countries who are embracing the challenges of this new technology. I was in New York to hear many of the scientists make their presentations at the *2nd International Stem Cell Conference* at the Academy of Medicine, organized and directed by Dr. Taylor's colleague, Dr. Warren Sherman. Both Dr. Sherman and Dr. Taylor played active roles as speakers and moderators of discussion throughout the two-day event. "When you realize how many millions of people are in dire need of assistance to continue their lives, and can grasp the potential that has been unlocked by cell therapy for the heart, the possibilities are staggering. The rate of progress and success are remarkable," stated Dr. Taylor.

Helping the Body Repair Itself

"When we started this journey in about 1989, it was a novel field; we did not really understand the concept of stem cells at the time. We did know myoblasts were 'reserve' cells that made new muscle. There was a learning curve; and we now believe that literally every tissue in the body has its own set of stem or progenitor cells within it. What I think is pretty remarkable is that for most of our lives our bodies are capable of repairing our tissues, if there are enough stem cells present, and providing the injury is not too catastrophic. In other words, we are finding out that virtually every organ in the body has some capacity for self-repair. Our job is to exploit that, to make it work longer and better, even in the face of catastrophic injury or illness." According to Dr. Taylor, the following approach is the one they focus on at the University of Minnesota:

1. We, as scientists, need to determine which cells will work best in the repair of a particular organ.

2. We then need to provide either the right cell or recruit the individual's own cells already present in

the body, for the prescribed task.

3. We must provide (empower) these cells with the right signals (the right cues or directions) to guide them, and then literally step aside and let nature take over.

"Therefore, our job as scientists will be to give the body the tools it needs, which at this point, I would argue, would have to be the right cells for the job and then to simply get out of the way and let the body do what it is capable of doing naturally – repair."

A Little History

Dr. Taylor continues, "In 1998 we published a seminal paper that showed we could transplant cells into the heart and improve function of the previously damaged heart. We were lucky enough to be the first people to accomplish this; and necessarily our studies were in animals. What turned out unexpectedly was that in just two years from our publication, independent clinical studies using the same cells began in Europe. When you realize how long the process usually takes to evolve, the way this took off was pretty amazing. We did not expect the studies to move nearly so rapidly. Our goal and intention in the early years was to first see if the concept would work. If it did, our plan was then to go back to our pre-clinical studies and do more in an attempt to understand more fully how it actually functions."

"We learned very soon after releasing our findings that we were a little naive in not anticipating two fairly immediate responses: (a) The number of patients who would contact us because of the enormous impact the information would have and (b) how quickly it would be moved forward by the clinical community. Even though our intention was to go back to the drawing board to better understand the technology in greater detail, the wheels were already in motion. Interestingly, as fate would have it, this unexpected momentum has given us the opportunity to answer questions both clinically and pre-clinically at the same time. To be candidly honest," added Dr. Taylor, "we still don't fully understand everything about it today — which also possibly means we haven't had the opportunity to make it the very best we can. Admittedly, when you don't fully yet understand a new science (even though things are moving forward well), you have to remain ever vigilant. Obviously, we do not want to do any harm to any patient but instead try and improve (his/her) quality of life. A vast number of these patients have no other remedies available. I think what we are developing with adult stem cells is bringing a wonderful opportunity to offer these advanced patients some viable options. WHAT I HAVE MAINTAINED ALL ALONG IS THAT MYOBLAST IS THE BEST FIRST GENERATION CELL PRODUCT. These cells can even produce molecules that cause blood vessels to grow and thus provide their own sustenance to continue living."

Now, besides the supportive words of Gandhi the doctor keeps on her office door, there is also a greeting card that has particular meaning for her. The card's caption reads, "Trust Your Crazy Ideas." Our interview time was running out just as Dr. Taylor was about to share one of those crazy ideas she and her colleagues had been working on first at Duke and now at the University of Minnesota. It would be several months later while attending the Inaugural Conference of the *International Society For Genomics, Proteomics and Cellular Therapy* at Scottsdale sponsored by the Arizona Heart Institute, that I too, as a guest, along with the gathered body of distinguished world leaders in stem cell research, would hear and see actual proof and early results, of one of those "crazy" research ideas. Dr. Taylor's presentation *Cell Based Repair: Putting Vascular Back in Cardiovascular* emphasized how the right cells, given the right instruction at the right time, can actually enhance the body's own ability to heal. It was amazing to see how these "intelligent" cells can be directed to intervene against heart disease at its very source, at it's core within the artery. The early study results Dr. Taylor presented would seem to indicate atherosclerosis might one day, (perhaps in the near future) be ameliorated where it actually begins and progresses—within the artery. This discovery is HUGE!

Can Stem Cells Neutralize Atherosclerosis?

Obviously heart disease is a disease of middle or advanced age, not found (except in certain rare genetic form) among the young. Therefore based on the sequence of transition, it would seem to make sense for the public to accept heart disease as a natural consequence of aging. To the scientist, the answer is far more complex and lies somewhere in the principal of supply and demand. What the average person accepts as normal, scientists may find clearly abnormal and seek to develop an understanding of how to alter the end result. That is why laymen are laymen and scientists are scientists.

The Role of Progenitor Cells, Atherosclerosis and Aging

Dr. Taylor along with colleagues, Pascal J. Goldschmidt-Clermont, M.D., Frederick Rauscher, M.D. and other team members from Duke University, Division of Cardiovascular/Medical Center in Durham NC had earlier pursued this aging phenomena in regard to the development of atherosclerosis in the aging population. The researchers would seek to better understand the role of this deficiency as it relates to the causation of heart disease and what could possibly be identified to interrupt that degenerative process. A process we have tended to accept as inevitable normal aging.

I asked Rauscher to explain. "Vascular progenitor cells (VPCs) come from the body's bone marrow and give rise to endothelium and other components of the blood vessel wall. VPCs are important to repair portions of the blood vessels that are damaged from stresses such as high blood pressure, high cholesterol and oxidative stress. We hypothesized that with aging there is a decreased supply of VPCs to repair the damage at the blood vessel wall, thus tipping the normal balance of injury and repair. With reduced VPCs in number and or quality, the body's chronically stressed arteries are not able to be repaired fast enough and atherosclerosis (plaque buildup) ensues."

Here again would be another classic case of cellular production breakdown brought about by an aging body's inability to meet supply with demand. So the question these scientists at Duke would hope to answer is what would happen if they found a way to help balance the supply of VPCs in keeping pace with the demand the aging arteries would require and therefore interrupt the damage and birth of atherosclerosis. A very worthwhile challenge to be sure. The potential here is exciting, now all the researchers had to do was find a way to prove their concept. Could they in effect, (using VPCs) alter the aging process within the arteries? More importantly could they in fact neutralize the arterial damage of atherosclerosis? To demonstrate this said Dr. Rauscher, we would take VPCs from the bone morrow of both young and old mice. To initiate the study the researchers would have to recruit very special little mice.

Because the normal lifespan of a mouse is a year and this study of atherosclerosis would focus on an aging mouse, this experiment would have to study a 6 month old plump, "midlife crisis" type mouse!

The researchers were looking for a little mouse who would not have a problem in submitting himself/herself to eating a very high fat diet for the following 6 months. No *Jenny Craig* Plan here. So the call went for volunteer mice. Needless to say the response for volunteers from the mouse community was enthusiastic and immediate. What vermin would not love to eat a diet that would be comparable to what our teenagers would be getting if they ate nothing but fast food and pizza for six months? Six months, according to the researcher is about middle age for a mouse.

Dr. Rauscher explains. "To demonstrate, we took VPCs from the bone marrow of both young and old mice. Each of the two groups were independently pre-dispositioned to develop severe atherosclerosis. However, the young healthier mice, because of their youth, (even though pre-dispositioned) had not yet developed the disease at the time we harvested their cells. Their healthy vascular pro-genitor cells said Dr. Rauscher, were protecting their young arteries. The old mice were now for the following six months placed on a high fat, high cholesterol diet con-sisting of more than five times the average cholesterol.

One group of mice were given the cells from young donors, while another group of mice were given the cells from the older animals. The cells were given six times, once every two weeks.

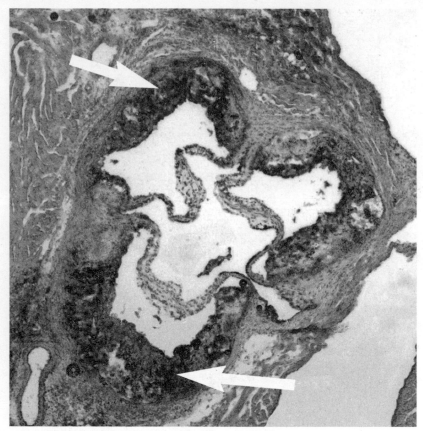

*Fig. 2 Dark area denotes advanced plaque in an older mouse artery before VPC treatment.

What Did the Study Prove About Aging and Heart Disease

"At six months, these mice, when their bone marrow cells were taken had developed much atherosclerosis. At that point we removed various arteries for analysis. In each of the artery locations tested there was significantly less plaque when the mice received bone marrow cells from young animals. In fact, when the bone marrow cells

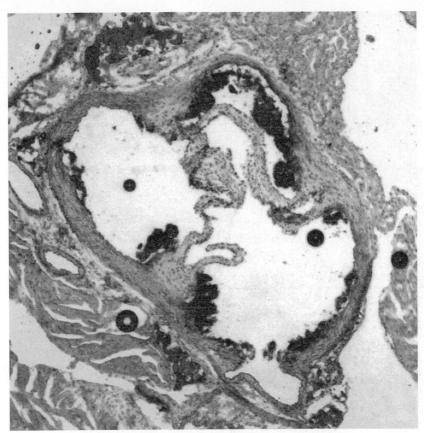

Fig. 3 Note: Plaque is almost totally dissolved after treatment with VPC cells from a young healthy mouse.

came from old mice, the plaque was the same or even worse than if no cells had been given at all. Therefore we concluded that the cells responsible for vascular repair become deficient with aging, resulting in atherosclerosis. However, what the study demonstrated was that the disease could be slowed down by giving supplemental vascular progenitor cells to animals as they age. In addition we showed that vascular repair by progenitor cells could attenuate atherosclerosis even in the presence of ongoing vascular damage (high cholesterol)."

*Fig. 2 & 3 By special permission, Circulation 2003; 108:457-463 TITLE: Aging Progenitor Cell Exhaustion and Atherosclerosis. Authors: Frederick M. Rauscher, MD; Pascal J. Goldschmidt-Clermont, MD; Bryce H. Davis, BSE; Tao Wang, MD, PhD; David Gregg, MD; Priya Ramaswami, BE; Anne M. Pippen, BS; Brian H. Annex, MD; Chunmig Dong, MD; Doris A. Taylor, PhD. Images on page 458.

Dr. Taylor on Gene and Cell Therapy: Present and Future

"This is a field just coming of age. We have an opportunity for the first time to treat the underlying issue that is a problem for tens of millions of people worldwide, repairing dead or damaged heart cells and blood vessels. The potential is great and yet we need to continue to learn from the treatments that have gone before us; treatments like gene therapy, asking what worked, what didn't work and how can we generally improve the therapies.

"There are many aspects of gene therapy that parallel cell therapy and still others that don't. We can learn a lot from them. For example, we have to do a better job of providing genes a target; we can't put genes into 'dead' scarred regions of the heart and expect them to work, they need to be able to target live cells to be active in the body. But if we can find the right targets, they can begin to have powerful effects. Cells are more forgiving. "We seem to be able to put cells in an injured heart and get an effect. Still with both cells and genes, it appears that they know exactly what to do if we give them the right cues and place them in the right environment. However, it seems to me that cells are the ultimate gene therapy, providing all the genes in one little box — a cell. They appear effective, at least to some degree, in an injured failing heart. I believe an issue we need to consider, is matching the right genes or cells with the right patient, at the right time. It may be that one cell type is better after someone has a heart attack and another cell type is better if one has heart failure. We are still learning. But what we do know, is there are a lot of patients with cardiovascular disease or peripheral vascular disease who just don't have any other options. These new treatments offer these patients a huge degree of hope that they haven't otherwise had. It's a great time to be doing this work, we can hopefully actually begin to change the way medicine is practiced and patients are treated. FDA-approved cell transplantation safety studies are currently in progress and the favorable evidence is mounting and is encouraging. The studies are moving forward with both bone marrow and myoblasts with almost no serious complications, even though the patient-base is often a very ill population."

Guiding This New Science Responsibly Forward

In 1977 scientist Dr. Andreas R. Gruentzig, developed the first catheter for angioplasty and performed the very first angioplasty procedure ever. We delve into more of his interesting story in the chapter on angioplasty. What is notable however is that Dr. Gruentzig resisted all early attempts by the media to publicize his discovery until he had the necessary time to perfect it. So concerned was he that a mistake could jeopardize the magnificent potential his discovery held for saving lives. As with any exciting breakthrough in medicine there are those who would take advantage. I think an excellent example of this might be what happened when cosmetic surgery first became an exciting and lucrative field. Certain physicians who were not really qualified began to exploit patients and the science by performing complex procedures without having the benefit of a comprehensive, dedicated and proper study. Some reportedly had attended a weekend seminar or watched videoed procedures to prepare themselves for surgery. As a result, many patients were disfigured and some even died. This wanton lack of professionalism brought the industry a black mark and negative traces that still unfortunately remain. Their unprofessional conduct ushered in a loss of confidence and subsequently altered plans for many potential patients. Dr. Taylor, as a pioneer of this newly emerging stem cell technology, candidly shared her insight in a desire to help lay responsible groundwork for proceeding forward.

She expressed her concern during my interview, "This is an exciting field. For better or worse that means everyone wants to do it, do it first and tell it to the press. What that can lead to is people jumping in to do clinical trials without having the basic training and understanding of what is involved. That means sometimes even the leaders in the field still have a lot to learn, at the same time as they begin to treat patients. I think it is absolutely critical that we move this new field forward quickly, but safely and responsibly, in such a way as to continue to bring hope to patients doing nothing to distract from the good work being done. What that means, is we need to understand the cells and their impact a little better. We also need to better understand for which patients, different cells might be appropriate, and answer some basic questions that remain, as to how, in the deepest sense, the cells actually work. We don't yet have all the answers but if we are going to bring the patient the best opportunity to capitalize on the hope this field holds, we continue to need to do more science; research is leading the way."

The professor also expressed her feeling that this is a critical time and it is important that the field judiciously choose the right clinical trials. "If we, as a field, enter into a wrongly-designed, very expensive clinical trial, those wrong choices can impact the hope of countless patients praying for their miracle. There is a need for the trials to proceed, but wisely, based on all we've learned to date." Why? Because, according to Dr. Taylor, "there is nothing worse than the dashed hope, the opportunity lost, progress squandered and the field set back. This field really has the potential to change the way medicine is practiced. Because it does, it is important to move it ahead as quickly as is safely possible while maximizing the potential for patient benefit. That will necessarily require discussion between scientists and clinicians. We must have basic science in place to explain the things we are seeing clinically and to respond to clinical challenges. If there is something a physician sees that they don't fully understand, they can't just go back and experiment. We do not experiment on people. Basic science has to step in. Likewise, we need to translate new ideas to patient care. We have identified the hope and now what we want to do, is go back, understand it more clearly (as was our original plan in 1989) and make it even better. Then, and only then, can we do what I've dreamed of since I was small, we can change the world – at least for patients living with heart disease."

Is the Industry Embracing Stem Cell Heart Therapy?

Five years ago, there were only 4 or 5 people like Dr. Taylor speaking about adult stem cell therapy before the American Heart Association. Last year the number increased to somewhere around 150 presentations and already this year, 25% of all the speeches at the AHA have been about stem cells for the heart. Also, according to Dr. Taylor. "Phase one and two trials are proceeding well in both the US and in Europe. The FDA has formed a new panel which goes by the name CBER (Center for Biologics Evaluation and Research) and the NIH (National Institutes of Health) is creating a special cardiovascular cell therapy trials network. This should answer the earlier question as to "how well the profession is embracing this new technology?" The attendance for Columbia University's *2nd International Stem Cell Conference* in New York sponsored by the *Cardiovascular Research Foundation* (CRF) had a more than 100% increased attendance over the previous year and the attendance for the coming year promises to be much larger. Further, the first ever, *Proteomics, Genomic, and Cellular Technology* conference sponsored by the Arizona Heart Institute in 2006 was highly successful, drawing leaders worldwide.

CHAPTER 4

Arizona Heart Institute
Cell Programs

*D*r. Nabil Dib, Chief of Cardiovascular Research at the Arizona Heart Institute, believes, "Clearly based on this new stem cell therapy, this is the way medicine is going to treat congestive heart failure and heart attacks in the very near future." Dr. Dib has successfully altered and converted previously scarred dead heart tissue to living functioning cells!

This institute has now had the benefit of more than 4 years of follow-up on the first patients to receive skeletal myoblast stem cell transplantation. Myoblast cells are adult cells taken from the patient's own thigh muscle, cultured in a dedicated laboratory and transplanted by minimally invasive intracoronary injection through the patient's femoral artery to the damaged portions of the heart.

"We have," says Dr. Dib, "after numerous clinical studies in human subjects over a period of time clearly and conclusively demonstrated that we can now definitely convert the damaged myocardial scarred cell to a healthy normal cell, through myoblast cell transfer."

Theoretically, these initial results completely refute previous medically accepted doctrine that there can be no hope of rejuvenation for hearts damaged from heart attack. What is critically important is that after more than four years into the trial the safety issue surrounding myoblast stem cell treatment has been effectively demonstrated and documented. With the benefit of hearing from actual patients whose heart health has been dramatically revived by the new cell procedure, you will be in a better informed position to make your own decision as to the viability of this new stem cell treatment.

Dr. Dib explains, "The four year trial was designed as a two-armed study, the first arm was designed to prove to the satisfaction of the governing agency certain provisions. The study Proof of Concept was:

A. Prove the cells we isolate from the subject can actually survive using muscle skeletal myoblast.

B. Prove we can expand these cells in the laboratory.

C. Prove we can transport the cells to the damaged scar tissue of the patient's heart.

D. Prove these cells survive and form myotoubin, myofiber (muscle cells and fibers)

E. Prove they, in fact, do express slow twitch protein necessary for long term heart function.

Protocol and Parameters of the Study

The study would be divided into 2 Arms with 12 patients in each Arm.

12 patients in Arm one will receive myoblast skeletal stem cell treatment.

12 patients in Arm two will not receive cells but will receive medication.

24 patients in total.

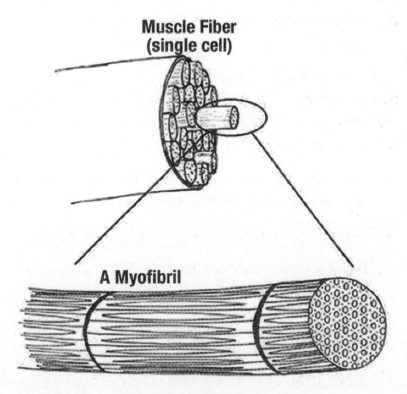

Fig. 4 Skeletal muscle fiber.

The first group of 3 patients to receive 30M cells.

The second group of 3 patients to receive 100M cells.

The third group of 3 patients to receive 300M cells.

The fourth group of 3 patients to receive 600M cells.

This first phase of the trial will complete in August 2006. Apparently the study results have been well received by the FDA. The government agency has just sanctioned the opening of 7 more stem cell heart trials nationwide.

"The qualifications that each study patient would have to meet would be important to the study's success. According to Dr. Dib, "The patients we would choose would actually be patients advanced in their disease and waiting for heart transplantation. The hearts of the patients would be qualified by testing with a technology called microscopy (mi-cros-co-py). The most conclusive accurate analysis of the patient's myocardial condition would be determined by applying histological (his-to-lo-gical) analysis. In our combined opinion at the Institute, we had believed that this would be the strongest and most conclusive evidence of the condition and perform-ance ability of the patient's heart."

"In each of these patients we would add additional pro-tection by implanting an LVAD (left ventricle assist device) to help maintain the patient's health by increasing func-tion of the left ventricle. We would add the device at the same time we would be implanting the patient's cells. It is important to note that each of the patients chosen had already been diagnosed with ischemic cardiomyopathy and had suffered one or more previous heart attacks. When finally a donor's "harvested heart" became available for the patient, we replaced the patient's natural heart with the donated heart. We would then proceed to do the histology and evaluation on the diseased heart, which we had just replaced. This is the heart into which we had earlier transplanted the cells from the patients own thigh muscle," explained Dr. Dib.

RESULTS: "Clearly, visible documented evidence in all cases that the cells were able to not only survive—which would answer the first Proof of Concept study question— but these cells did also successfully create new tissue— answering the second important proof of concept question. Beyond that, these new cells aligned parallel to the heart's healthy tissue, later adding to the heart's ability to contract. Importantly, yes the question of expression was also answered favorably as to the survival of the fatigue slow twitch protein, required for long term survival."

"We know," says Dr. Dib, "that the scar tissue has only 20% of the normal blood supply compared to what the normal cardiac muscle has. That would be a significant lower rate of deficiency of 80%. We realized that those myoblasts, which our study was utilizing for repairing the damaged myocardium, would be extracted from the skeletal muscle. The skeletal muscle resides in an area of low producing oxygen. Importantly to our concept is the fact that we know medically that the scar tissue cannot repair itself but the skeletal muscle cells can and do bring the necessary repair." I had spent time with Dr. Dib on a few occasions and had expressed an interest to be an observer of an actual stem cell transplant procedure at the Arizona Heart Institute. I had that opportunity in May 2006. I had the distinct impression that the minimally invasive procedure, once given final FDA approval, will be readily adopted by interventional cardiologists in their practices to the benefit of all of us. I asked Dr. Dib, why in particular, did you decide to concentrate on the skeletal cells? "The major reason why we chose to use them was because we believed they would survive in a low oxygen state which they would have to do to be viable for the heart. These cells are predetermined to be muscle and cannot provide any other kind of tissue. Herein lies the scientific rationale for muscle cell myoblast cells for myocardial damage. The histology that was derived from analyzing the patient's diseased hearts after transplantation with the new donor heart accomplished our obligation in meeting the requirements of the FDA guidelines." Then these cells are autologous? From the patient's own body? "Correct," answers Dr. Dib. There will be many references to the term *ejection fraction* (EF), throughout the book, particularly in determining the before and after affects of stem cell transfer. Because of its importance in determining cardiovascular health, this is a good time to explain the relevance and ultimate importance of the ejection fraction as a marker of determination of one's cardiac condition. The left ventricle (chamber) supplies the oxygen carrying blood to the body. How well it is able to pump in order to fulfill it's appointed task is generally read and determined by either an echocardiogram (ultrasound), MRI, (magnetic resonance imaging) fast CT (computed tomography imaging), or a nuclear treadmill. A normal ejection fraction is between 50-70%, which means 50-70% of the blood is being ejected to the rest of the body. When the EF drops below 40 heart failure is considered the diagnosis.

It was Time to Qualify and Recruit Patients

The institute would choose and enroll 24 initial patients for the safety trial.

Criteria for Qualification:

1. Patients must have sustained a previous myocardial infarction (heart attack).

2. The first 12 subjects to be chosen would have an EF of 30%.

3. The second group of subjects would have an EF of less than 40%.

4. Each of these patients in final selection would have been candidates for bypass surgery and had previously sustained significant heart muscle damage.

5. Our objective would be first to perform the bypass surgery, opening the compromised arterial flow, and

then, to simultaneously inject myoblast skeletal cells into the diseased scar tissue of the patient's heart.

We would use an escalating number of cells graduating from 10-20-30-100 and 300 million cultured cells. Significantly, the safety factor remained consistently positive throughout.

What you are about to read will put a smile on your face, very possibly the hope of new life for your heart and the vision and promise of the better life you have only thus far dared to dream.

Seeing is Believing: Meet the First Patient

Sixty-two year old Samuel Cohen may be described as a no-nonsense former New Yorker, now a retired dentist living in Arizona. "I knew when I received the news that the prognosis for someone with congestive heart failure is one to five years duration, I must have had angels looking over me, because had I not been afforded the opportunity at Arizona Heart, I would probably be dead today. Make no mistake," said Sam, "it is between you, your maker and the team that has been assembled on your behalf that gets you through."

Dr. Cohen had come to Phoenix, Arizona to build his dental practice in 1987. All was going well, according to him, until December of 1993. It was nearing the end of the year that he began experiencing a lot more discomforting tightness in his chest during his regular walks. He was aware that something was amiss. As he explains, "I had this overall feeling that something regarding my health just wasn't at all right. It concerned me enough that I decided to pay a visit to the Phoenix Baptist Hospital where they ran preliminary diagnostic tests." The results demanded and justified an immediate angiogram. Sam continues, "The procedure informed the cardiologist that there was a 99% blockage in my left main artery. Before I would leave the Hospital I would require and undergo surgery for a five-way bypass." Sam's message to all of us would be listen to your own body and submit to regular checkups.

Patient's Medical History

A little of Sam's familial and personal health history: Sam's father died at age 62 from a heart attack and Sam had been a pretty dedicated smoker. As he says, "I was always a Lucky Strike man, I had smoked for about 31 years. If you are wondering what my cholesterol was in 1998, the total cholesterol number was 222 mg/dl."

Coincidentally, according to a national survey, the average total cholesterol for people admitted to hospitals with a heart attack was not as high as one might expect. The number ascertained by the survey was not 285, 260 or even 240. No, the average total cholesterol number was 220 mg/dl. Dr. Cohen's low-density lipids, LDL (the bad one), were at the time measured at 156, with a high-density lipoprotein, HDL (the good one), in the low range of

41. Therefore, there was a combination of risk factors that most likely had contributed to Dr. Cohen's heart disease: Smoking (which is still the number one rated risk factor), low HDL and high LDL cholesterol. Two more risk factors one could add to the profile, as with any man of 62, would be age and gender.

Sam goes on, "Now in 1995 (two years after the 5-way bypass), my cardiologist, while listening to my carotid arteries with his stethoscope, heard a 'bruit.'" A bruit is a swishing sound alerting the physician that a blockage is forming in a carotid artery leading to the brain. A follow-up Doppler ultrasound confirmed the obstruction was large enough to warrant an endarterectomy (en-dar-ter-ec-tomy), a surgical procedure to clear the neck arteries. The American Heart Association guidelines suggest an endarterectomy when the occlusion in the carotid reaches 60% or more. If, however, your condition is asymptomatic, (exhibiting no symptoms) but found to be at least 70% blocked you may still be a candidate for surgery. It may sound a little confusing but if it turned out that your carotid artery was not more than 50% blocked and you were exhibiting symptoms, your cardiologist may still recommend surgery.

Sam explains, "During the time from 1995 to 1999 I had been seeing my cardiologist every four months and was having annual stress tests. Also, during that four-year period, because of ongoing stenosis (plaque buildup), it had been necessary for me to have several additional stents implanted in the original bypass grafts. The bad news would come in 1999 when the cardiologist said—'Sam, we've got a problem. There is significant blockage in your circumflex artery.' The doctor informed me that this is the artery that feeds the back of the heart. I was thinking, no big deal, we can do this. Here we go with another stent like I already had installed several times before. This time, however, it would not be business as usual. It would not simply be another trip to the catherization lab for an automatic 'quick fix.'" As Sam clarifies, "The cardiologist did not feel he could be successful in stenting the circumflex because of the specific location of the blockage. His concern was that plaque debris could become displaced during the procedure blocking an opening to a native vessel, resulting in a major heart attack."

According to Sam's cardiologist, if the accumulated plaque blocked the native vessel, Sam could not be a candidate for a bypass. His doctor made an appointment for him at the Mayo Clinic to seek a second opinion. Dr. Cohen recalls, "Another cardiologist, after reviewing my records told me, 'Sam, you are between a rock and a hard place.' He discussed that he could try and place a stent in the circumflex, but he shared the very same concerns, as did the original cardiologist. Well, as you might imagine," says Sam, "I am not a happy camper, at this point. I gather up all my films and make my way to the Arizona Heart Institute."

Do You Have a Miracle for Me?

"I met with an interventional cardiologist who also happened to be the Chief of Cardiovascular Research at the institute, Dr. Nabil Dib, who analyzed all the information, the scans and the earlier blood work I had brought with me. He informed me that on a positive note, I had a good deal of collateral circulation going for me. [Collateral arteries are small vessels the body has developed to provide a natural bypass past an occluded artery.] This was a good thing. However, even with the benefit of the collateral circulation, several months later in early 1999, Sam still experienced his first heart attack. "It was Dr. Dib who found a way to position a stent where the two cardiologists earlier had deferred."

Months later during one of my visits with Dr. Dib at the Arizona Heart Institute, I asked him how he had found a way through the blocked artery to place Sam's stent? He explained he had actually gone in through one of the collaterals.

Dr. Cohen continues, "Now, sometime between six months and a year later [Sam wasn't quite sure], I am sitting on my sofa and suddenly become aware that my heart is radiating. My wife immediately drove me to the Institute and I am diagnosed as having acute congestive heart failure. This is not a heart attack that I am having but acute heart failure. The hospital kept me overnight, in the morning, Dr. Dib performed a procedure to install an intra-aortic balloon pump (IABP). [A procedure in which a balloon is fed up through the femoral artery into the aorta.] The way they explained the procedure to me said Sam, was that when the heart contracts, the balloon will keep the blood from traveling back into the pulmonary artery and into my lungs. In just 24 hours they had reversed my immediate condition of acute heart failure. To me it was mind-boggling. I was out of the acute congestive heart failure but in general, I was still theoretically considered positive for heart failure. Dr. Dib explained to me that the circumflex, in spite of the stenting, was still more closed than he had imagined. The left main artery had been 99% closed so he also opened it for me at the same time he stented the circumflex. At this point the doctor said, 'Sam, we need to do something more for you.'

Dr. Deitritch, the founder of the Arizona Heart Institute is also a cardio thoracic surgeon and interventional cardiologist Intimately involved in all aspects of the Institute's procedures. He personally withdrew the cells from Dr. Cohen's thigh muscle. The harvested cells were then cultured in the lab until they escalated in number to 300M cells and injected into the area of dead heart muscle in Sam's heart. This was done at the same time as they did the bypass surgery. Note: Sam needed two procedures— the bypass surgery to open blood flow and the second procedure to implant stem cells to heal the heart now in heart failure.

Dr. Cohen added, "Over the next two years they performed the regular diagnostics to measure my progress. In the beginning it was every 3 months, PET scans, MRI's. EKG's, echocardiograms and whatever tests were needed to document my progress for the research." Soon after the surgery (Sam did not recall the actual months) the increase in glucose activity, representing cellular growth, became obvious and a good sign that the cell transplant was stimulating regeneration. "I went back to work as a dentist following the July 4th holiday. I had taken two months off work following my circumflex, bypass surgery and stem cell transplant on May 6, 2000."

Dr. Cohen was the very first patient to benefit from Arizona Heart Institute's heart stem cell program and after a full six years since his procedure he continues to do well and describes himself as very grateful. See Sam's remarkable actual before and after MRI results in the color illustrations section Figure 11.

An Alternate to Endarterectomy

There is an alternative procedure to endarterectomy surgery now available had Sam been diagnosed and scheduled for surgery today. Two FDA approved stenting devices provide surgeons an alternative way to stent the carotid artery at the point of severe narrowing. These new stent procedures also carry their own set of risk as does standard endarterectomy. The results of two studies reported in Journal of *Vascular Surgery* in 2005 and *The New England Journal of Medicine*, respectively, earlier in

2004. There was no difference in study outcomes when the two approaches were evaluated side by side. It therefore becomes a choice between you and your physician as to which procedure to apply, stenting or endarterectomy surgery.

A Heart-to-Heart with Duane Gutcher

Duane is today a very grateful man 66 years of age. He explains that at the time of his heart attack he had been seeing his doctor for routine visits and physicals. Because his cholesterol was borderline (as he described it) he had not required medication. He experienced his heart attack on 6-20-99. When I asked about his family history he could not recall there being heart disease within his family, except to say his mother died of congestive heart failure at 80 years of age. At the time of his attack, Duane was a very active individual who swam regularly, hiked frequently and enjoyed bike riding with his wife. He explains, "During one of these mountain hikes on a Friday in June, while I was engaged in strenuous climbing, I felt warm, light-headed and noticed my skin feeling clammy. Basically, I just didn't feel right. The discomfort was pronounced enough to dissuade me from continuing the climb and my wife and I cancelled our hike and returned to our motor home." Duane recalled that he remembered thinking he had never felt quite this way before. Other victims of heart attack, whose stories you will read, described a similar ominous discomfort prior to their attacks.

Still, at this point of discomfort, Duane wasn't thinking heart attack— there would be time enough for that realization later. As a matter of fact, two days after his Friday symptoms completely vacated, a Sunday afternoon would mark the day of his crisis. He goes on, "Mrs. Gutcher and I had returned from our morning church service, ate lunch–then feeling weak and tired I went in to take a nap. It would be approximately an hour later that I awakened from my sleep with a growing tightness in my chest and feeling very light headed. I laid down on the floor seeking some relief. The weakness I had been feeling was going to put me on the floor whether I wanted to be there or not."

Now, for the very first time Duane actually knew he was indeed having everyone's worst nightmare, a heart attack! Here was one of those cases that you often hear about where one is comforted by the sudden disappearance of symptoms and sees no need to see a doctor. No, Duane had not realized the Friday night symptoms were a warning sign of what was about to happen two days later on that Sunday afternoon. Some heart attacks hit strong and others begin slowly. This slow onset is one reason why half of all the people wait too long, actually an average two hours before calling for help. This is a major contributing reason to why 250,000 heart attack victims each year do not survive to get to the hospital. Duane continues his story, "By the time the paramedics arrived I was in excruciating pain that had literally brought me to screams." Anyone who has gone through this valley knows what Duane was talking about. Here is what could be described as a two-ton gorilla jumping on your breastbone like a trampoline.

I don't think Duane would mind me sharing with you that "it flat hurt like #$%! I was sure thinking I may be very close to meeting my maker." As you will read in additional patient interviews, a spiritual element presents itself. Whether you are or aren't a religious or spiritual individual, you realize your life is suddenly out of your control and you are very inclined to seek a higher power whatever your persuasion.

Hospital, here I come! The hospital's ER was about a 3-mile drive and they began the tests immediately upon Duane's admittance. Several years ago a drug called (tPA) had been developed and fortunately for Duane, they administered it to him due haste. Originally, (tPA) was a drug developed to break up clots that are involved in brain attacks. It has since become a drug to be used similarly to breaking up a clot formation in a heart attack. The longer it takes for a clot to pass through a blocked heart artery, the more damage is sustained by the myocardium. As doctor Kumar Ravi always reminds his patients, "time is heart muscle."

Fortunately for Duane, they must have identified him as a good candidate for the drug. There is a window of about 6-8 hours when the drug can work its magic following a stroke or heart attack. Therein lies one very good example why someone's symptoms should not be overlooked. Here is a very good reason for seeking immediate medical attention rather than waiting to see your regular doctor two or three days later. It may be now or never!

Duane tells me, "It was verified that indeed I had experienced a heart attack. I was placed in ICU and remained there for 3 or 4 days. To my knowledge they had not at this point in time diagnosed the degree of damage that my heart had sustained. I was released with the advice to report to my physician and to seek a cardiologist's care."

Remember, Duane had been an avid hiker and bike rider before his incident, and now he describes himself as "not nearly the person I was before the attack." That is a feeling that no doubt many readers who have experienced a single or multiple heart attack will relate to. It is certainly understandable. Other diseases that diminish one's strength and overall health may take years in their devastation, therefore one has time to gradually adjust to the reality. With a heart attack, the change is not spread over time and gradually accepted. It is, instead, immediate and profound. An active, athletic, vital individual can overnight begin to feel (in their own mind) like a diminished person of lesser stature and value. One is faced with the reality that the tasks one could perform just yesterday, today cannot be done at all or at least not as well.

Duane explains, "I had reconciled myself at this point to

just going about life in slow motion. Any exertion tired me and the order of the day was—don't push your luck. I was taking 5 and 6 naps a day." Duane would attribute a great deal to general fatigue but also a good amount of blame to being depressed over the entire crisis and a sinking lack of hope. At this point Duane described his appearance as being horrible and colorless, and as generally experiencing a total lack of energy. He simply did not feel at all well. Basically, Duane spent hours just sitting. Fear and depression are real and present dangers following a heart attack and Duane was no different in his reaction in not wanting to be active. Finally a little over a month after his heart attack, an angiogram would be performed to determine the degree of damage and to define what actually had caused Duane's heart attack. The procedure found a 90% blocked coronary artery and a significant blockage in another. Both arteries would receive medicated stents. Today, the stents would most likely have been one of the newer improved drug eluting stents.

The Prognosis

Duane was told his ejection fraction following his heart attack was a low 34 and that he could not expect to see his condition improve. There were (as the physicians saw it) two options available. One was to have two pacemakers installed. The damage must have been significant because Duane was forewarned that this first option may not work at all. "They told me the chances of success did not look very good." The second option, (and this would be the first time Duane heard of it) would be a new procedure called stem cell skeletal myoblast transplant. "After having the new procedure explained, without giving it a second thought, I said, what have I got to lose? I had already decided before I even got to the Institute that if I were accepted into the program I would give it a shot." Six weeks later Duane would have an interview with the two principal doctors, Edward Dietriech founder of the Arizona Heart Institute and surgeon and Nabil Dib, Interventional Cardiologist and Principal Investigator for the stem cell transfer project. "The procedure was explained to me and the elimination and critical analysis was begun to learn if, in fact, I would be accepted as one of the first patients to have this procedure."

"I am believing this sounds all too good to be true. On 2-21-05, six weeks after the cells were drawn from my thigh muscle to be cultured, the cell transplant took place." Were you fearful or reticent going into this experimental surgery? I asked Duane, he responded, "No, I had no fear at all and I just believed this was going to be successful."

POST SURGERY: "They did the implantation about 10:00 am and they kept me awake that first night as they were monitoring me, giving me echocardiograms, EKGs etc. By the third day I just noticeably felt better. It was unreal! I really wondered if I might be experiencing a placebo effect? I asked Dr. Dib if I could actually be getting benefit so soon? He explained that even after just 3 days the cells are already fusing and beginning to work. Within a full week I could not deny the marked improvement. When they checked me with echocardiogram my ejection fraction had jumped from the low 30's prior to surgery to an amazing 53 with the stem cells." I found myself duly impressed as I remarked, Duane, that is a pretty normal EF for anyone. "Now," explains Duane, "about two months later when I went in for my consultation, having had a very successful nuclear stress test, I was simply elated as were the doctors with my results and how good I was feeling. I told them I was now able to do just about anything, I didn't have to slow down and I was swimming once again. I was able to go for 1 mile walks a day and I know this may be difficult to believe, but I actually raced Loretta, one of Dr. Dib's assistants up 4 flights of stairs and actually outdid her!"

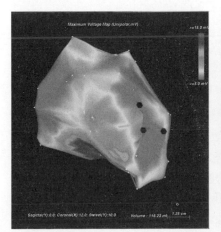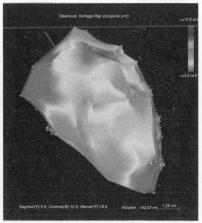

Figs. 5 & 6 Duane's before and after 3-dimensional Noga Mapping scans show amazing and conclusive heart repair. See color images Figs. 8 and 9.

It is now a year later and Duane continues to do extremely well. He adds, "It's almost like a miracle, a day and night difference. I go days without feeling a need to lie down, whereas before I needed to take several naps a day."

Five Heart Attacks and Doing Fantastic

Matthew, how are you feeling? "I just feel fannnn-tas-tic!" came Matthew Plummer's reply. Could I take you back to the beginning Matt and ask you what your life was like before your first heart attack? "Well, I was work-ing full-time for Lockheed Martin Goodyear and was enrolled three-fourths of the time at DeVry Institute of Technology. Life was good, my wife and I were doing well and I was looking forward to graduating."

THE FIRST HEART ATTACK, Matthew explained, "It came in 1997 and happened while I was attending one of my classes at DeVry. I had been very involved working and studying for exams. On this day the exam had major importance and the stress level was notable." Some peo-ple having a heart attack describe intense pain in different parts of the anatomy. In Matthew's case, it was through-out his entire body. Was he having a heart attack? "Well" said Matt, "I didn't think so but then I admit I had not been to a doctor in years and was not aware of my cho-lesterol or other risk factors. No, at this time I did not con-sider I was having an attack. I knew, of course, something that I sure didn't understand was happening."

As with many of the people I have talked to about their heart attacks, they mention putting out a call to their higher power. Matt was no different. "I talked to the man upstairs. I asked him what was happening to me, what was going so wrong?" Anyone who has survived their heart attack will tell you there is that fear of the unexpected—the anticipation their heart may cease to beat in the next instant. They are right. Self-sufficiency and self-reliance at this moment become only buzz words for a self-motivational seminar. Your life is in someone else's hands and you are clearly not in control! Yes, there is a spiritual component to having a heart attack. Matt was not in denial, he just wasn't aware of the symptoms of a heart attack. His total focus and concentration had been on work and furthering his education. He added, "I excused myself from class and went home early. I could barely make it home." As Matt described the trip, "I had to wrap my arms through the steering wheel. I tried massaging my temples to relieve the pain, took an aspirin [which ultimately might have helped get him through this first attack] passed out, and awoke the next day feeling a lot better and continued working." Wow, what a day Matt!

Heart Attacks, Two and Three

About a year later Matt is still working at Lockheed. He has just graduated and as he explains, he was not under undue stress as he had been during his first heart attack two years earlier at the DeVry Institute. "This time I am at home when an elephant stomps on my chest!" Not really, but that's how heart attack pain is often described and that is exactly the expression Matt related to me. Matt explained, "One afternoon while I am home watching television, my wife and her friend had just left the house when I have another very intense heart attack. This one is as strong as the very first one I had at school. When my wife returned home I was already at the hospital." This time, Matt drove himself to the hospital. It was fortunate for him that he made it. While he is being evaluated for heart attack number two he has a third heart attack. Matthew Plummer is informed by the ER attending physician that he is not only having a heart attack but his EKG has indicated that he has had two before this one. This is number three! He later learns that his total cholesterol just happened to be an alarming 586! An angiogram was performed. "I was not happy to hear the ER doctor explain to me that my arteries are smaller than average and with the identified amount of plaque buildup, I was not a candidate for angioplasty and stents to open the narrowed arteries." Matt recalls there was also no mention of the possibility of open-heart surgery as an option. As Matt shared, "This guy's beside manner wasn't the best. He really upset me by telling me at that very inappropriate moment that my career was over. I should quit my job and seek a new line of work." To add to Matt's distress (for whatever reason) the doctor chose that moment of great anxiety and fear to tell Matt he could expect to continue having attacks in his future, which actually turned out to be an accurate prognosis, as we will soon see.

Driving Oneself to the Hospital?

Under the same circumstances most people having a heart attack would probably not have made it to the hospital. They could have become snarled in traffic, taken the wrong route, very possibly passed out, or moved to sudden death. Every year heart attacks and strokes cause drivers to not only kill themselves, but also innocent victims as passengers in oncoming vehicles. According to Prediman (PK) Shah, Director of Cardiology at Cedars Sinai Medical Center in Los Angeles, your chances are better with a paramedic or ambulance than having a friend or family member drive you. As Dr. Shah asks, "What can a non-professional do for you if your heart stops en-route to the ER? A paramedic has equipment to re-start the heart and the knowledge to intervene in preserving someone's life," concludes Dr. Shah.

Of the 370,000 heart attacks in a given year 250,000 do not survive for a full hour following the attack. In medicine they talk about "the golden hour" in which a patient must receive medical attention and become stabilized. When you speak about cardiac arrest and heart attacks, the time is limited to minutes and possibly seconds. Many die in the first few minutes, so the earliest call to 911, according to the American Heart Association, may be your strongest chance of survival. Most people, not real-

izing the symptoms, delay in making the initial call, thinking the chest, jaw or shoulder pain, shortness of breath or
heavy perspiration will pass. This time of delay is vital in
the response scenario. The quicker you, as a patient, get
medical attention, the greater your chances of minimizing heart damage. It costs a great more many lives every
year when an EMT arrives on the scene a few minutes too
late. So many times the 5-10-30 minute or two-hour
delay in the patient moving to action and making the
phone call, contributes to their demise.

In the case of stroke, a person's brain becomes affected
if they have been deprived of oxygen for only 3.5 minutes.
The average national time for ambulance, fire department
or paramedic response is 5.7 minutes. In many individual
cases, because of excessive traffic, an incorrect home
address or mechanical breakdown, the time may be 12-18-
20 minutes or even longer. Further, there is a systemic
problem and disparity between EMT or ambulance
response time in rural communities as compared to that in
cities. There are tangible reasons for this discrepancy. There
are many outlying communities with limited resources who
because of budgetary restraints must rely on volunteer
emergency personnel. This is not meant to be disrespectful
to these dedicated volunteers but distance and time to
mobilize can cause major delays in response from the time
of the first phone call. If you have someone with you to
perform CPR in the interim, you will do better. However,
regardless of the statistics, in Matthew's case he did the

right thing for Matt—he survived!

A year and half passes and Matt learns, through his brother-in-law of the groundbreaking work being done at the Arizona Heart Institute. An appointment is set and Matt is scheduled for his first office visit. At the time Matt's doctors explained to him they were doing all they could but outside of an attempt at controlling his cholesterol, their options were limited. Matt is following his doctor's advice, modifying his diet, taking medication including cholesterol lowering regime and following a plan of treatment. He described his mental state of mind as being very depressed.

Heart Attack Number Four and Counting

Matt continues, "I meet with Dr. Harvey Hecht and began working with him, having all the tests that I had not had before—stress, echoes, every test imaginable. Basically I was put through the diagnostic mill. I cannot say enough about the thoroughness of the care I received." He recalls his time on the treadmill to be short, approximately 4.5 minutes and the pain in his legs he described as severe.

"Dr. Hecht wanted to evaluate what was going on in my legs," explained Matt. Claudication or intermittent claudication are two related conditions in which the blood flow through the legs is diminished as a result of plaque buildup in the leg arteries. Claudication is a result of peripheral artery disease (PAD). Intermittent claudication occurs when one is walking even short distances but is relieved if the subject sits for a time. The first type is more advanced and the pain is chronic whether one is walking or not. A Doppler ultrasound is the usual test for determining one's degree of carotid obstruction. Matt received a more critical evaluation as he was given a dye injection as a tracer agent and the vessels leading to the legs from the groin area were found to be occluded. An angiogram procedure was successfully performed and four stents were implemented two in each artery leading to the left and right legs. Matt immediately felt the improvement. Angiography and stenting are not procedures used exclusively for the heart. Matt described the improvement, "Before my legs were stented I could barely walk, but under doctor's orders following my procedures, I began to walk everyday. One block each day for the first week, two blocks each day for the next 5 days, then a mile, then two miles a day. Feeling so encouraged I went out and bought myself a bicycle and began a 7-mile a day program!"

Heart Attack Number Five

As fate would have it, a year later Matt would suffer his fifth heart attack. Ironically he had just entered the Arizona Heart facility and is seated in the lobby when it happens. Matt recovers after his hospital stay and returns home. He quits his job at Lockheed Martin Goodyear following his graduation from DeVry and joins MCI WorldCom.

Hearing About Myoblast Stem Cell Therapy
October 2003

Dr. Hecht has now left the Arizona Heart for other commitments and Dr. Shakur is administering to Matt. At this point in time Matt had decided to pursue a life-long, unfulfilled desire to live in Florida. "Before I would relocate to Florida, I decided to see my friends at Arizona Heart one more time. I wanted to be completely evaluated before making my move to the Southeast." Reading the results of Matt's new tests, Dr. Shakur was of the belief that Matt might be wise to undergo bypass surgery and to do it before going to Florida. A subsequent meeting was set at the institute and as Matt explained, he and his wife were seated when Dr. Nabil Dib and nurse practitioner, Sean Kane, entered the room. They had already conferred with Dr. Shukur concerning his recommendation for Matt to have bypass surgery.

"My wife and I accompanied the two gentlemen to a viewing room where they proceeded to show us films of what was actually going on with my heart. The front and back sections of my heart were literally immobile and the only pumping movement was at the bottom of the heart with some light movement on the sides. My heart was enlarged from the additional pumping it had been required to do to compensate for the damaged sections. You didn't have to be a trained cardiologist to get the picture. My wife and I obviously did not like what we saw. The bypass procedure I would require would be a four-way bypass. The doctors showed us collateral vessels (natural bypass arterioles), which are blood vessels that form on their own forcing blood pathways around the blocked arteries," just as in Dr. Cohen's case. This natural process of angiogenesis is what very well may have been keeping Matt alive for the prior few years. "I didn't know until then," said Matt, "what a collateral artery was."

If you have ever wondered how someone who has been told that he or she had a 99% or 100% blocked artery can still be alive, the answer might lie in the fact that in such cases the body had developed collateral arteries around the occluded vessel. Those individuals who have been physically active or involved in regular exercise may develop these collaterals more readily than others. Matt's ejection fraction was 26. Fifty-five and higher is normal. Matt's EF by any standard was at a decisively low number.

He was looking at his chances, his options. "Do I want to go ahead with bypass? As it stood, I knew my outlook was poor and I for sure valued my life, I remember thinking, if I could even have another five years." Matt recalls his feelings, "In my mind I am at the best facility and have the best doctors I could have anywhere. I'm thinking how every minute of everyday is valued, I am very grateful after all the heart attacks to still be alive and I decided, yes, If I am accepted as a candidate I would do it!"

In an earlier chapter we discussed how heart attack victims frequently experience depression along with their illness. In Matt's case he now realized he had been somewhat in a state of depression all the way back since his very first heart attack. He explained that the depression had intensified with each of the four attacks that followed. The negative information given him by the attending ER doctor at the first hospital still haunted him. As he explained, "I was shot in the foot by the demoralizing kick I got from the first ER doctor."

"Most people are not lucky enough to survive the first MI and I had 5. Many times through the previous years as one attack happened after another, I had wondered why the man upstairs had not taken me. Well, I am glad he didn't as I am very happy to be alive and now, I was believing a door was opening, thanks to these two physicians Dib and Dietreich, who were standing there saying 'we're going to fix you!'"

"The doctors had shown my wife and I the filmed results of the earlier evaluation and pointed out the four arteries that would have to be bypassed. Sean set me up to begin the further evaluation and if I qualified, I would begin the cell capture process in which my own cells would be cultured and prepared in the laboratory for implementation into my heart at the time of the bypass surgery. I would be notified approximately 4-6 weeks after the muscle cells would be drawn from my thigh muscle. The doctor leaves and Sean, the nurse practitioner, begins to explain the myoblast stem cell two-year study (which at that time would have begun almost two years earlier). Sean patiently explained the highly involved technical information to us in a simple presentation, which we were able to understand. I was aware that heart transplants and recovery are long term and the chances of rejection remain very high. As Sean explained it, these are my own muscle cells being cultured and transplanted and I would not be facing rejection. This almost sounds too good to be true. This would be a miracle! Immediately upon making my decision to go forward I felt like a weight had been taken off of my shoulders. Here I am about to be given this miracle surgery by the best guys I could have and they are believing I am going to have a changed life. It is too good to be true and yet here I am as if I had truly been lead."

Day of Reckoning Arrives

"I get the call informing me to be at the Arizona Heart Hospital 5:00 AM the next morning. The surgery went well as expected, and now a few days after the surgery I was home recuperating—lying on my back watching television and all of a sudden, I notice movement in my chest area beneath my shirt. My chest is literally moving up and down like I hadn't seen it in years. My heart was beating and pumping normally! What a feeling. Wow I'm thinking! This is a fantastic sign. My heart is pumping as strong as it had been before my five heart attacks." I could hear the excitement in Matt's voice as he relived the experience. Matt observes, "This was a healthy heart functioning as it had years earlier prior to the first heart attack!" Two more weeks would pass before Matt would be re-evaluated to monitor the progress at the hospital. During the first month he would go in about once a week. They were [according to Matt] administering all the ultrasounds, echocardiograms, etc. to evaluate my progress. "I believe it was the third week's visit when they told me my ejection fraction had already increased and was now at an amazing 40% compared to the low of 26% prior to surgery."

UPDATE: More than a year after the surgery Matt informs me and he would like you to know, that he has not had a single symptom or setback! Matt is walking everyday, his eating habits have changed, he is on medication and working full time. He is very grateful and in his words, "I'm feeling fannnn-tastic!"

Joe Gasser, a non-smoker and non-drinker, had been in real estate and development for almost 50 years, was 65 years of age and in semi-retirement, when he started to become noticeably fatigued. Joe is now 72 and looking back, explains at the end of April in 1997 he was aware that something just wasn't right. The tiredness he was experiencing had come on him 7-10 days prior to his heart attack. Joe, shares, that to his knowledge at the time, he was actually in pretty good shape. "That was until I went to a highly respected facility in Mesa to undergo a physical examination." I asked Joe, as I had several of the other patients, if there had been a familial history of heart disease. Joe replied that he had no significant memory of any—he was the first.

"I was given an EKG at the facility and sent home with the instruction to return the following day. I went home, relaxing after dinner, became involved in reading." Joe's heart attack was not a slowly building event telegraphed by radiating pain in the arm, jaw or chest. As Joe explains, "It hit hard that same night, the pain was so severe that I was all but paralyzed. In spite of the fact that I was hardly able to move I did get myself to my bed where I put in a call to my doctor, who called in a prescription for nitroglycerin. I had a friend pick it up for me and the nitro did bring some relief." I asked, "You weren't told to call 911? No one suggested that you have someone other than yourself, drive you immediately to the ER after having experienced what certainly appeared to be an obvious attack? "No," said Joe "the following day I drove to the ER myself and was given a test and immediately following the procedure the doctor instructed me to get myself to the hospital ASAP! The suggestion was that I make a decision to either drive myself to the hospital or have them order an ambulance."

At this point in Joe's story, I wonder if you, like me, are somewhat amazed at the advice Joe had been given. First, after describing his symptoms initially why was he not told to call 911 rather than waiting for nitroglycerin to be delivered by a friend? Second, why was he given a choice of driving himself to the hospital? "As soon as I arrived at the hospital," said Joe, "they prepped me, performed an angiogram and promptly inserted a stent. I am not told much about my condition—at least not that I remember—but I know that I am not comfortable with the cardiologist and seek a second opinion as to my condition and prognosis." Joe had been given medications, which he explained brought him some relief but mentioned that his heart must have been quite severely damaged. He had learned that his ejection fraction measured by an echocardiogram was very low at 19." Obviously you must have sustained a major attack! "That fact," says Joe, "was what I became more aware of as time went on. I began working with a different cardiologist who continued to monitor my progress over the following months. At one point in 2002 my EF actually dropped to an even more significant low of 15." 15! Joe, that is in the basement.

"At this point the new doctor in no uncertain words said, 'Joe, you should be dead!' At this time 75% of my heart was not even functioning and I was surviving with only 25% of the heart's viability."

Joe continues, "My cardiologist suggested I see the team at the Arizona Heart Institute to learn if I would be considered for a dual procedure to install both a pacemaker and a defibrillator. [A pacemaker to regulate the

heartbeat and a defibrillator as a fail safe method to literally shock one back to life if the heart stops in cardiac
arrest.] "This would be my first association with Arizona
Heart. I met with a Doctor Ruzio who implemented the
devices. They worked great and I found myself much
more active and even reconstituted my swimming routine each day." In general, Joe said, "I felt very good."
Most patients will tell you there is some added sense of
security knowing they have the benefit of these backup
systems monitoring their heart functions. Joe goes on to
recount that, in December 2003, he became aware of
what a defibrillator actually sounds and feels like when it
is rudely activated. "I had been lying on my stomach
when it activated and it almost knocked me out of my
bed. I literally awoke with a jolt!" For the purpose of illus-
tration, an implanted defibrillator offers the same function as do the lifesaving "paddles" we so often have seen
deployed on TV medical drama shows like ER or what we
might have seen depicted on *Gray's Anatomy*. The procedure literally shocks one back to life when the heart has
straight-lined. The shock has the kick of a mule! After this
experience, Joe's cardiologists at Arizona Heart had decided it would be an advantage for Joe to replace his current
two-line model. Medtronic, a leader in cardio devices,
had found in a six month study of 450 patients, those
patients with the newer 3 line model were able to walk
further, exercise longer and in general do better overall.
This advanced model is the one Joe received to replace
the older two-line defibrillator.

I ask, "Joe, what have the doctors told you about what you might expect from this point forward?" Joe replies, "I am told that as the heart gets larger from the damage I will eventually go into congestive heart failure leading to eventual cardiac arrest. It is at this point that Doctor Ruzio suggests a meeting with Dr. Dib to learn if my case might be a consideration for the new myoblast stem cell transplant. It is now early 2004. I let a couple of months pass and then decided to call the Institute to find out if in fact, I might qualify as a candidate for this new procedure. It is now the beginning of 2005 and I was put through a thorough and extensive testing schedule. The word finally came down from Dr. Dib that yes, I would be given the option."

Would you describe your mood as nervous, anxious, apprehensive? "I had nothing to lose and I had definitely done my homework. Another consideration that in finality gave me the confidence to proceed was how pleased and comfortable I had become with the professional courtesy and respectful way these doctors at the Institute related to me. You know how often times you are almost intimidated in discussing your health with a doctor? You almost feel like you shouldn't have even brought up the question." We both laughed as we anticipated how many of you reading this story would relate from personal experience. "Not so with this team of physicians" says Joe, "They took whatever time necessary in answering my many questions and concerns. Particularly those I had about the various tests I was to be put through. Another point that I am sure weighed heavily in going forward was what my previous cardiologist had told me in suggesting the Institute for the pacemaker, when he said this was probably the only chance of survival I had left on the table. It all came together and I felt very comfortable in making my final decision."

"It has been a relatively short time since my procedure and I am definitely feeling better but as you might understand, I am not jumping up and down on a trampoline." Joe's progress from a low ejection fraction of just 15 prior to the surgery to one of 24 three months later is encouraging and should continue to improve over the next six months. Joe is once again swimming and bike riding each morning. To those who err on the side of caution in regard to heart disease, being quick to action is prudent practice, proven so in Joe's case.

A New FDA Approved Trial for the Arizona Heart Institute

In mid 2006 the FDA gave approval for a first of it's kind trial to address acute myocardial infarction using special bone marrow derived stem cells. This new bone marrow study will initially accept 20 patients within 30-60 days after they experienced their heart attack. The current ongoing myoblast skeletal stem cell trial did not have this 30-60 day window but accepted patients whose heart attack had happened long before they began treatment.

When Symptoms Occur, Before the Ambulance Arrives

At the outset of symptoms, taking an aspirin is the recommendation from the AMA. This is not a time for a 40 mg "baby aspirin" but a 325 mg tablet or its equivalence of 4-80 mg tablets according to the advice. The object here is to have the medication dissolve into the blood stream as soon as possible. If all you have available is *time released* coated aspirin, chew it, thereby breaking the shell. Coated aspirin is designed to not dissolve until it enters the small intestine 30 minutes to an hour or so after ingestion, someone experiencing the attack will need the therapy immediately. Aspirin mediates against platelet aggregation, the process that forms the clot. Even though the symptoms do disappear [as they sometimes will] you may not be out of the woods. You very possibly were having an attack or very close to one. You may have been given a temporary reprieve but this would not be a time to allow yourself to become complacent. What you were experiencing still requires an evaluation for cardiac enzymes and further examination to determine if you were in fact having a heart attack. The narrowed coronary arteries would of course still remain compromised and there may be another episode lurking in the wings. Seeking immediate medical attention at the onset of symptoms is the prudent advice any cardiologist would give. No one would want to experience a heart attack as Duane and Matt recounted in their stories.

CHAPTER 5

Acid Reflux
or a *Heart Attack?*

*T*housands of people each year innocently mistake their heart attack symptoms for heartburn and mistake heartburn for a heart attack. As the King in *The King and I* musical would say, "it is a puzzlement," particularly in diagnosing women's heart attacks. How many women each year are sent home from the ER or from the physician's office with a purse full of antacids, only to learn after the fact, that all along, her symptoms were not a case of upset stomach or acid reflux but warnings of heart attack. It would be a vital life saving bit of information if there was a fail safe way for you and me to accurately determine the difference. Unfortunately there is not. But here are a few possibilities to consider. Mind you, these are not warnings that one can etch in stone. Nothing is as accurate as blood tests to measure enzyme levels and cardiac markers to determine a heart attack in progress. Nevertheless, here are a few simple questions to ask yourself if you are trying to determine the difference between a heart attack and indigestion:

- What were you doing just prior to becoming aware of the discomfort?

- Had you been over exerting yourself just before your symptoms began? Were you pushing yourself beyond your endurance or conditioning? "Weekend Warriors," as example, really push their luck in chancing a heart attack as physical activity increases their risk dramatically. Dr. Satyendra Giri found in his study that heart risk is ten times greater among people who have maintained very low physical activity and who have several risk factors in their profile. In general there is a reported 5.9 times risk for heart attack among subjects within one hour of having high physical output, according to an 1800 patient study done by the Institutes of Health.

- Were you involved in an emotionally charged argument or discussion? Old family resentments, rivalries and personal issues explode during arguments and heated exchanges. If alcohol is involved it only exacerbates and fuels the fire. Studies have found that the risk of heart attack or stroke increases immediately after such emotional conflict.

- Do you have a history of heart problems, particularly angina? You may have been given a prescription for nitroglycerin, which will relieve the symptom temporarily but will also help you define the problem as being heart related.

- Is there pain radiating in the arm, the jaw, the chest or

shoulder? Obviously, take any of these warnings very seriously as indications of heart involvement.

• Are you displaying symptoms in very cold weather? Narrowed arteries can constrict even more in the cold, bringing one to crisis. Heart attacks increase every year during the winter months—a reported 34% higher number happening during peak winter months compared to the summer when they are at their lowest numbers.

• Did the discomfort begin soon after you had finished a heavy fat meal?

Here are a few reasons why it is so difficult even for the physician to determine the difference between indigestion and heart attacks. To begin with, the symptoms of both heart attack and acid reflux can be very similar. Given a 50-50 tossup between the two ailments, one is likely to choose the lesser of the two evils. Consider the following discussion of how discomfort after a heavy meal may be easily misdiagnosed. Triglycerides (circulating blood fats) can "spike" to dangerous levels immediately following a single fat meal leading directly to a heart attack, according to M.D., Ph.D., FACC— Michael Miller, Director of Preventive Cardiology at the University of Maryland. Studies have found an increase of 20% in reported heart attacks during a holiday such as Thanksgiving. The irony is that indigestion legitimately can follow dining as well. The question must still be answered, is it definitively a heart attack or merely indigestion? To further complicate matters, nausea, a symptom of indigestion, can also be one of the warnings of a heart attack, particularly among women. So one can see how difficult it is to always know the difference between the two conditions.

Another type of pain, often misdiagnosed as indigestion, is a form of heart pain called angina pectoris that heightens when the heart is not getting enough oxygen carrying blood. The key that may be helpful in determining the difference between the two dysfunctions is angina is usually felt deep within the chest and is described more like an ache, pressure or even tightness in the chest as opposed to a burning sensation, one often associates with indigestion. Can someone be comfortable making a decision based on the symptom? Not really, because heart attack is also frequently described as a burning sensation in the chest as well. It becomes apparent that there is no easy answer, particularly when one's life might hang in the balance. No time to make a mistake.

The very classic case to make this point, regarding problems of diagnosis, is what happened to Ed Bradley of *60 Minutes* fame. As he related his story on the *Larry King Show*, Mr. Bradley had been having chest pain and went to his doctor who gave him antacids after diagnosing his condition as acid reflux. Ed took the pills for about two weeks, as he explained, and then informed the doctor that the pills were not bringing any relief. He was about to go to the Middle East on assignment and wanted to have his health situation resolved before leaving. His doctor prescribed a different medication for acid reflux and Ed left on his overseas trip. The pains continued and when he returned to the states another doctor performed an endoscopy procedure, looking inside Ed's stomach. As Mr. Bradley came out of the anesthesia he learned, to his surprise, that he did not have acid reflux but that his pains were more than likely, heart related. He went back to the first doctor who suggested a stress test and left the office with a prescription for nitroglycerin tablets with the instruction to put one under his tongue when, and if, he experienced pain. It was time for this patient to seek an opinion of a cardiologist and fortunately Ed Bradley chose one of the finest doctors in the country, Dr. Valentin Fuster, former President of the American Heart Association, now with Mt. Sinai Medical Center in New York City. To make the story short, Dr. Fuster, according to the *60 Minutes* reporter, said, "If you were my brother I wouldn't let you leave the hospital tonight." In the morning, Ed Bradley went into surgery and had a five-way bypass!

No Pat Answers Between Heart Attack and Acid Reflux

As you see there are no pat answers, there is no certain way of knowing for sure which of the two conditions, acid reflux or heart attack you are experiencing. Damned if you do and damned if you don't. Any physician who tells you otherwise is only rendering an educated guess. If this characterization of an "educated guess" were not true, there would not be hundreds, if not thousands, of cases a year, where even the ER has misdiagnosed these same symptoms. The major concern for you as a patient may be in the "golden hour" of needing a paramedic or an immediate trip to the ER. What are you going to do? Be safe or sorry? Say to your wife or husband, "Let's sleep on it and if it doesn't go away by morning we'll see the doctor?" The morning never comes for thousands of people each year in the same predicament. It's your call.

CHAPTER 6

Columbia University
Stem Cell Program

*D*r. WARREN SHERMAN, Director of the Columbia University Medical Center in New York City, directs the clinical stem cell therapy programs within the Division of Cardiology. Dr. Sherman brings a wealth of experience and an interesting perspective to this new technology, as someone involved with the very first skeletal myoblast cell transfer ever done (without surgery) in a human being and as an established interventional cardiologist and Associate Director of Mt. Sinai's Catheterization Laboratory in New York. With his team, he performed the very first cellular transplant for congestive heart failure. This first ground breaking task was accomplished in the Netherlands, May 25th, 2001, and involved transplantation of skeletal myoblast cells from the patient's own leg muscle to her heart. The minimally invasive procedure was performed with team members Dr. Kumar Ravi of Phoenix, Arizona and Dr. Peter Smits of Rotterdam. While at Beth Israel Hospital in New York, Dr's Ravi and Sherman had previously been looking at the role of gene therapy for coronary heart disease patients when they became involved with a stem cell transitional study that eventuated (developed) into a clinical study. Dr. Sherman joined Mt. Sinai Medical Center in 2001, working with Dr. Fuster.

Making Medical History

The landmark event in 2001 was described as the first ever non-surgical endovascular case performed on a human to augment heart function. An accomplishment that inspired Patrick Serruys M.D., PhD., team leader and professor of Interventional Cardiology at Erasmus University to comment, "This may be one of the most significant developments in the history of treating heart disease patients." Now, having participated in and directing studies currently in progress at Columbia University Medical Center in New York that concern both myoblast and bone marrow applications for the heart, who better than Dr. Sherman to address a few fundamental questions?

Myoblast or Bone Marrow?

"Both types of cells are, most commonly, autologous [from the person's own body] and homogeneous [having similar characteristics]. Recently, however, bone marrow cells from a donor have been used. Myoblasts are immature muscle cells," Dr. Sherman explains, "That are extracted from a muscle in the upper leg. They are destined to become mature muscle cells when needed —that is their one and only purpose. Bone marrow cells on the other hand are a very diverse population of cells. Although they are being used and studied for heart repair they also have a great degree of versatility and capacity for assisting in the treatment of other diseases. Bone marrow cells are used in the replacement of red blood cells, white blood cells, and platelets. For decades they have also been used to treat patients with leukemia and lymphoma, as well as for more than 70 other diseases. Myoblasts, as effective as they are proving to be in heart repair, do not have the same broad scope of versatility."

Is There a Consensus Forming in the Industry?

Dr. Sherman continues, "The majority of data from the research community so far reasonably and strongly suggests that the heart muscle can increase in strength with skeletal myoblast transplantation from the leg muscle." In contrast Dr. Sherman explains, "The data accumulated from bone marrow cells at this point in time indicate that if there is a condition that involves insufficient blood supply to the heart—as in cases of ischemic coronary heart disease—blood marrow cells can indeed strengthen a weakened area of the heart. They specifically accomplish this by helping to increase blood vessel supply resulting in improved heart output and better heart function." Dr Sherman is precise in adding that this derived benefit would be the result of having enhanced blood vessel flow to the heart and not the result of having added more muscle, as would be the case with myoblast therapy." With emphasis on the word "possibility," Dr. Sherman discussed how these bone marrow cells may be helpful in performing a unique treatment that might actually repair blood vessels, especially the lining of these vessels. Dr's. Taylor, Hare, Sherman and Dib have also acknowledged this new role for cell therapy.

An Exciting New Area of Repair

According to Dr. Sherman, "Within a broader population of cells as one might expect with bone marrow, there are cells that serve to repair various components of blood vessels and especially the vessel linings. When a person experiences a heart attack there are signals that are released into the blood from the site of injury. These signals are picked up by the bone marrow and other reservoirs of cells. They call out to repair cells and particularly to those involved with vascular repair to migrate into the circulation. Here they seek out the actual site of injury to begin a process of rescue and repair. One could think of it as a distress call to 911 or a Mayday call for help!"

Dr. Sherman continues, "That process is enacted in the acute heart attack setting. Months or years later, after the heart has formed scar tissue, a different type of cell is needed. These autologous host cells are drawn from the patient's own leg muscle, isolated, cultured in a special dedicated laboratory specifically for this purpose. Once they are cultured to the right number of cells, [in a matter of weeks] they are then transferred via catheter to the heart. Dr. Ravi and I had been involved in helping the Bioheart Company develop their catheter. Incidentally this is the same company that also cultures and prepares the cells we use for the transplants."

I ask, "I would imagine many of your patients would wonder how you control the actual deployment of the cells? For instance, how do you know how deep to go into the muscle?" Dr. Sherman replies, "we measure the thickness of the heart muscle prior to the procedure. Our catheter has an adjustable needle, which enables us to control the precise depth into the muscle. As an example, with yesterday's patient we used a depth between 3 and 4 mil-

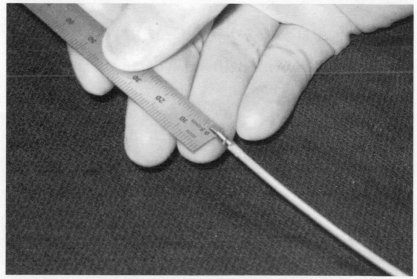

Fig. 7 Adjusting a predetermined catheter needle length

limeters." How do you determine the exact target area? "At this point in our current study we are only permitted to use low doses of cell numbers, the protocol is currently limited to just 6 injections. Even though a heart attack or attacks can cover a fairly large area, with our limited number of injections in this first phase permitted, we choose to inject at least for now, centrally into the overall damaged area. The FDA designed study began in 2003 with nine patients with a target of 50. "Significantly" said Dr. Sherman, "this would be the first FDA approved study using this type of cell for this population of patients and would be part of an ongoing multi-center investigation." During the first phase of the trial the Columbia team began administering smaller patient doses. As safety issues were monitored and as things progressed well, the second phase of the study begins to use increased therapeutic dosages.

Myoblast or Bone Marrow

Regardless of how well things seem to progress, there is always the voice of reason stating that, though the general feeling among a particular field of physicians and researchers is that they are developing a viable therapy, there is still no guarantee of success. No one knows for sure if the science will work long term. Having said that, Sherman believes that the opinion of most of the researchers in the field is that what they are implementing in the multi-center study will work and it will be proven that it works. Now, addressing the differences between the two types of cells Dr. Sherman explains, "fundamentally, muscle cells basically resemble one another and are limited in their prescribed ability to diversify. Bone marrow cells on the other hand, differ as they are from a very diverse population of cells. These bone marrow cells are homogenous and therefore could most likely provide additional purpose, in serving different kinds of diseases. Muscle cells are dedicated to one purpose while bone marrow cells have more versatility in their scope. In the late nineties we decided to direct our attention less in the direction of gene therapy for patients with coronary heart disease and more in the direction and potential of stem cell therapy."

I ask, "Can you share an example of where the versatility of one approach might provide a specific advantage?" Dr. Sherman responds, "when a condition exists of insufficient blood flow to the heart as with ischemic heart disease, the early studies have shown blood marrow cells can provide a solution by increasing blood vessel supply to that region of the heart. The patient's ejection fraction would be improved; however, the improvement would probably have resulted from the increased blood flow and not from strengthening the actual heart muscle itself." The benefit, as Dr. Sherman emphasizes, would be accomplished by a regeneration of the vessel as opposed to regeneration of the actual heart muscle, as with direct cell transplantation.

Wayne Meserve's Interrupted Flight

Wayne, a very articulate 56-year-old patient, was treated with myoblast cells in the first phase of the Columbia study. Consequently, in accordance with the FDA guidelines, he received a lower dose of cells than what would have been permitted in the second cohort. It was a year earlier in 2005 that Wayne had his treatment performed by Dr. Sherman. Wayne described his history and general condition prior to his heart attack as a profile that had no indication of heart disease. He was a runner and received a stress test every year as part of his annual physical. I might add here that Bill Clinton has said publically that he had aced his treadmills every year he had been in the White House and still had an open-heart 5-way bypass. Two prominent individuals whose deaths surprised a lot of people were Jim Fixx and the recent death of Dr. Lynn Smaha. Dr. Smaha was himself an interventional cardiologist and a former president of the American Heart Association. Fixx and Dr. Smaha were runners. In spite of their healthy habits each died of a heart attack. Dr. Smaha's death came while exercising in April 2006. It doesn't bring a lot of comfort to realize; presidents with all the best medical advisors and even knowledgeable members of the cardiovascular community still are at risk from heart attack.

Obviously, there are reasons for heart attack that avoid detection in the normal course of inspection. Wayne Meserve explains that he had always been conscious of his diet. Although in retrospect, he adds that he could have been a few pounds lighter. He was certainly not

obese or much overweight. When asked about his cholesterol levels he assures me that they were in the moderate
range with very good reported ratios. In further support
of the low risk cholesterol issue is the fact that his doctor
at the time told Wayne there was no reason to treat him
for high cholesterol. This turns out to be a particularly
interesting case in that it substantiates the fact, 50% of all
heart attacks do happen to people with normal cholesterol. Rounding out his history, Wayne mentions that he
was being treated for mild hypertension (Cozar®) and in
general was a pretty active individual.

On October 20th, 2001 Wayne, accompanied by his wife
and dog, was piloting a small plane enroute to their second
home in Maine. He explains, "About 20 minutes into the
flight, I became aware of an uneasy feeling. I'm just not feeling well. It was not the typical crushing pain in the chest nor
was it a case of jaw or arm pain." Wayne instead, describes
an aching in his left side. "I wondered what could be causing it?" Many of us having similar discomfort might have
dismissed the cause as indigestion, blaming it on something
we had eaten. Luckily for Wayne, he did not dismiss it. "At
this point in the flight, I informed my wife we were going to
return to the airport as I was becoming convinced that I was
indeed having a heart attack. When my wife and I arrived
home, I immediately took two aspirin as prophylaxis and
headed straight for the hospital." What Wayne said transpired at the hospital may not surprise you, having read
other patients' stories of misdiagnosis in earlier chapters.

The hospital claimed in their initial assessment that Wayne was not having a heart attack. If you think this misdiagnosis is unusual, it has actually happened literally hundreds, if not thousands of times. It happens more frequently to women at hospitals and even ER staff members have too often failed to recognize that a woman's warning symptoms are often very different from a man's. Frequently, as the statistics bear out, women have been sent home and incorrectly told theirs was a case of acid reflux or indigestion. Some of those unlucky women have actually died because of the misinformation, as we have previously discussed.

In Wayne's situation, he explained that he did not get properly diagnosed for 12 hours. We have talked about the "golden hour" and the adage *"Time is muscle."* The longer treatment is delayed in either a stroke or a heart attack the more damage can be done. Wayne would sometime later learn from his own cardiologist that his measurement of heart viability had now dropped to a low 22%. Wayne says, "The doctor did not actually come out immediately or directly with the information; he was however, fairly insistent upon impressing upon me that I really needed to be outfitted with a defibrillator, an ICD (implantable cardioverter defibrillator). The cardiologist shared with me the statistics associated with morbidity and mortality rates associated with a low ejection fraction. I had been doing my due diligence and had researched what it meant to have an ejection fraction in the low 20's and decided to take my doctor's precautionary advice."

"More than once I had engaged my cardiologist in conversation about my personal philosophy of life. I told him at my age it is not about just being alive, it is about living. Therefore I was willing to try anything, a promising clinical trial or just about anything short of a visit to a witch doctor. After hearing me repeat my wish on more than one occasion, my doctor finally said, 'Look, I know this fellow Sherman at Columbia in New York and yours is the kind of case he would be interested in as a researcher. He suggested I write to Dr. Sherman. I promptly heard back from the doctor and he proceeded to discuss the procedure with me. At that point in time I would become the second case in the trial, with only one prior case having been done by Dr. Sherman at Mt. Sinai Medical Center." Wayne did qualify for the procedure and six months after his stem cell myoblast transfer Wayne shared with me, "I am now feeling stronger and can do things with greater ease." Wayne's philosophy and willingness to take a chance to live a full and normal life once again had paid off. As Wayne explained, "I just refused to give in!"

There is one question that Wayne mentioned had never been answered: What had actually caused his heart attack? In his case, Ischemic heart disease, the most frequent cause of heart attacks, had been ruled out. The assessment was that it was not a typical case of a heart attack caused by narrowing of the coronary arteries [ischemic coronary heart disease]. Instead it was determined by his physicians that a plaque had ruptured in the left anterior descending artery (LAD). Based on the clinical evidence gathered from his attack, Wayne's case, absent typical coronary blockages from cholesterol buildup, would be best explained by the doctors as one of *Vulnerable Plaque.*

> *M.D., John Rumberger, Director, Healthwise Diagnostic Center in Columbus Ohio, Prediman (PK) Shah, Chief of Cardiology and Atherosclerosis Research at Cedars Sinai Medical Center, Los Angeles, CA along with M.D., associates, Daniel Berman, Matthew J. Price and colleagues, Paul Ridker, David Siscovic, Peter Libby and more than 20 other leaders in this field have defined the risks of this phenomena in their study, From vulnerable plaque to vulnerable patient: a call for new definitions and risk assessment strategies.*

(Continues in Chapter 7)

Vulnerable Plaque and *Inflammation,* *Major Risk Factors*

*T*he discovery and understanding of Vulnerable Plaque is a phenomenon that can explain how many heart attacks happen among people without history or obvious heart disease. Remember this fact that I have admittedly repeated several times in the book because what it says, is so 'right on point' and relative to the discussion. Fifty percent of all heart attacks happen among people with normal cholesterol? According to a report from the AHA, 80% of patients who are in recovery following a heart attack have unstable plaque located a distance from the original rupture. The report goes on to say, following an acute coronary syndrome, which would include heart attack or severe chest pain, there is a high risk of another coronary episode happening within the following year. According to the study's author Gilles Rioufol, M.D., Ph.D Associate Professor in Lyon, France, "We were surprised to find that almost four out of five patients present one or more ruptured atherosclerotic plaques besides the culprit lesion. In one out of eight patients all three main arteries were affected." There is apparently a large buildup of plaque in the inner linings of the arteries after such an event. It has now become apparent that inflammation within the arteries is a vital link to heart disease and heart attacks, exacerbating and heightening the risk of vulnerable plaque disruption and hemorrhage. When there is actual injury following a heart attack, inflammatory response is setup within the arteries. Secondary ruptures some distance from the initial site frequently happen within the months following the original attack. Coumadin (warfarin) or Plavix® (clopidogrel), as well as aspirin are helpful in minimizing damage from such a secondary event and recent studies have indicated longer is better for the use of blood thinners during the first year. Once a rise in inflammation is identified, measures can now be implemented to help control and modify the forces of inflammation that contribute to plaque vulnerability. This is why having a hi-sensitivity CRP test is a valued diagnostic. It is reported, that 500,000 people a year die from vulnerable plaque disruption. One person per minute falls to this type of heart attack.

Haven't you and I tried to understand how a famous athlete or someone we knew personally, who monitored his/her health, exercised, ate right, passed a treadmill test and still succumbed to a heart attack? Vulnerable Plaque disruption helps explain how this can happen and why one person with low or normal cholesterol might have a cardiovascular event while another with high cholesterol may not. Dr. Steven Nissan from the Cleveland Clinic, (President of the American College of Cardiology) in his earlier work with intravascular ultrasound (IVRUS) brought awareness and explanation of how vulnerable plaque manifests and causes attacks. Employing a tiny camera IVRUS (intravascular ultrasound) fed into the artery, cardiologists are able to now observe the plaque formation. Dr. Nissan established that coronary plaque in its construction is not all alike. The evidence shows that certain plaques are more susceptible to becoming dislodged than other plaques and in fact the larger more solidified calcified lesions may not (contrary to prior accepted belief) be the ones most likely to burst. The smaller more recently formed plaques, (less than 50%), often called "soft plaques," have now been proven more susceptible to rupture, leading to a heart attack. There are two basic types according to Dr. Nissan's findings. One presents with a large lipid core and a thin fibrous cap. The doctor explains that this type is very vulnerable to rupture. The second classification is even more dangerous. This type presents with a smaller body or core, but with a heavier cap; therefore, it is "top heavy" and even more prone to explode and rupture. Vulnerable plaque helps explain how someone previously appearing in excellent cardiovascular health can suddenly displace plaque that eventuates into a heart or brain attack. Cardiologists attributed Wayne Meserve's attack to vulnerable plaque.

Inflammation as Important
if not more than Cholesterol

Modern medicine even in the late 1990's concentrated on cholesterol as the sole reason for heart disease. Most of us are probably now aware of inflammation's role in heart disease and the studies that recognize it to be as important as cholesterol in determining who might be most inclined toward and destined for an attack. How many times have you heard of someone having a heart attack who had no family history of heart disease, who maintained very low cholesterol and who exercised religiously? You may be thinking of someone in your own family who had such an experience. The reason might lie in a silent increase of the inflammatory CRP marker. According to M.D., Paul Ridker of Bringham and Woman's Hospital in Boston MA, and Director of the Physician's Health Study, 25-35 million Americans are at risk for heart attacks from inflammation. Dr. Ridker's research helped enlighten cardiologists and general physicians worldwide as to how an inflamed endothelium (arterial wall) can provide an unstable base for cholesterol deposits to rupture and block an artery. The findings of the Physician's Health Study since the late 1980's began to bring attention to the role of inflammation. Dr. Russell Ross, from the University of Washington, had earlier attracted attention to what he identified as an impressive body of evidence strongly suggesting that atherosclerosis begins with damage to the cells that line blood vessels supplying the heart. The vessels narrow as the cells attempt to repair themselves, causing inflammation and this, in turn, attracts and traps cholesterol and immune system cells contributing to damage of the vessel walls. It was Dr. Russell who first identified cardiovascular disease as being not just a degenerative disease (as been previously known) but that heart disease, was also an inflammatory one.

Undetected Inflammation

Do you know if you or members of your family have an unidentified risk of inflammation in their cardiovascular profile? The information gathered from the Physician's Health Study opened a new area of research and understanding of how inflammation impacts one's risk of heart disease. The study also answered a question that had confounded medicine for half a century—why a person with normal cholesterol readings can still experience a massive heart attack? After investigating the risk profile of 1,800 physician participants, the Physician's study found that those subjects who had elevated CRP scores were at a 300% risk of having a heart attack over the following 6-8 years. Now, if a subject in the study had both an elevation in CRP and an elevation in LDL cholesterol, that combination brought a 500% increased risk over the same amount of time. Here again, I feel compelled to repeat the statistic one more time. Yes, CRP is a major reason 50% of all heart attacks do actually occur among people, with so-called "normal" cholesterol. In my discussion with Dr. Ridker for my earlier book, in which the subtitle happened to be *Inflammation, Cardiology's Newest Frontier*, Dr. Ridker explained some of the contributing factors that contribute to elevations in this all important marker. The identifying test incidentally, is called a high sensitivity (HS-CRP). Inflammation is a concern to women as much as men. In a report published by the journal *Circulation* of the American Heart Association CRP, when moderately to highly elevated levels among women, was found to increase women's heart attack risk 7-fold. The Study author who reported on the study findings was Dr. Oscar Bazzino of the Italian hospital in Buenos Aires, Argentina. Dr. Ridker established the current CRP guidelines for determining risk.

√ A score of below one as low risk.

√ A score of between 1 and 2.9 as moderate risk.

√ A score above 3 as high risk.

What can lower CRP? Aspirin was found in the Physician's Health Study to lower inflammation by 55.7%! Fish oil lowers it, as does exercise and loss of weight, cessation of smoking, anti-inflammatory medications and in several cases, steroids under close medical supervision. With the withdrawal of anti-inflammatory drugs like Vioxx®, Bextra® and Mobid® and the discrediting of others because of side effects, many are turning to the natural community for alternative inflammation fighters. [Inflammation as a measurement of heat can cause existing plaque to burst].

Low Grade Infections
that Inflame Artery Walls

The inner linings that surround the lumen (arterial opening) are the endothelium linings of the artery where the damage from free radicals and cholesterol deposits, various oxidative stresses, calcium, fibrin, smoking, inflammation and radiation contributes to atherosclerosis. In ischemic heart disease, these are the vessels where plaque forms, dislodges and occludes an artery creating the myocardial infarction or (heart attack) we all fear. Here is another area of ongoing injury, repair and the inflammatory response that has become a totally new focus of heart disease research and study in recent years. Included in the list of enemies to the artery walls are at least 3 low grade infections. Chlamydia pneumoniae (e) (klah-MID'e-ah nu-MO'ne-i), an upper respiratory infection that is usually first acquired in childhood. Even though the occasional lingering seasonal cough and associated wheezing will disappear, the infection becomes dormant. Unless one is tested and treated with appropriate antibiotics, it may continue to reactivate, inflaming arterial walls throughout one's lifetime. Bronchial asthma patients may also do well to have the blood test for this infection. Helicobacter pylori (HEL'eh-ko-bak"ter pi-LO'ri) is a second low grade infection associated with stomach ulcers and digestive problems, also now implicated with heart disease. A third infection is a viral infection called Cytomegalovirus, CMV (ci"to-meg"ah-lo-VI'rus). A study appearing in the *Archives of Internal Medicine* found of 700 subjects those with antibodies for CMV were at a 76% greater chance of having a heart attack compared to those who did not harbor the antibodies. If one has an elevation in HS-CRP, the physician needs to consider further specific blood tests to find the actual cause of the elevation. Is it attributable to gum disease, CMV, herpes simplex, chlamydia pneumonia, rheumatoid arthritis, polymyalgia, lupus, cancer, obesity or any other inflammatory source? Viral infections are much more difficult to treat than their bacterial cousins. If inflammation is truly as important or more important than cholesterol, the full set of risk factors must be evaluated. If one has a heart attack from either high cholesterol deposits or from high inflammation the end result is obviously the same.

Columbia's First Myoblast Stem Cell Transfer in the US

Jose Ramirez may be the quintessential, hard working New York family man. After having autologous myoblast cell transplantation to his damaged heart, the 46 year old said, "The main thing is—I am now going to be around to see my grandchildren grow up and my daughter graduate. No, I'm not going anywhere for a while." Jose's battle with heart disease began very early in his life after suffering his first heart attack at age 34. Over the next 14 years Jose would experience a total of 4 heart attacks—as in *f-o-u-r!* Looking back to his first attack, Jose recalls, "It was pretty scary, not like anything I had experienced before and something I sure didn't understand. Whatever it is that is happening—you realize you just don't have any control over it. I kept thinking this must be what people are talking about when they describe their event. I still didn't want to believe it. Heart attacks are not something I knew about or wanted to know about. I kept telling myself, they just don't happen to young guys like me! At least so I thought."

I asked Jose how this all began? "It was my typical morning starting off for work. I had stopped to grab a roll and a carton of orange juice, nothing out of the ordinary. I was apparently having symptoms, which I did not recognize as being heart related. I blamed the tightness in my chest as being caused by gas from acidity in the juice. As it turned out— as you will see, I was almost dead wrong. I tried to burp, thinking that would take away the pressure." Jose candidly explains that at the time of his attack he was smoking 3 packs a day of his favorite cigarettes. His total cholesterol in 2003, a little over 13 years after his first attack was still a whopping 293 with an LDL of 193 and an HDL of 41. He explains he is now at this time taking better care of himself. What his cholesterol profile would have been 13 and a half years earlier during the first heart attack, one could only speculate.

Jose continues his recollection. "At this point the (morning of my attack) the pain is getting stronger and I tell my boss I probably should get some medical help. I arrived at the hospital about 25 minutes later. They took the mystery out of my 'gas attack' when they flat told me the words I sure didn't want to hear. 'You are having a heart attack.' The doctors were surprised at my young age so they didn't want to do anything too dramatic." [Anyone having open-heart surgery at a young age might require a second open-heart surgery within a few years and there is only so much graft artery material available for additional surgeries. Using other measures available such as stents, medication, dietary modification and exercise has been considered the better course in the short term]. "I believe they felt they could control the future with medications, but they definitely told me I had to quit smoking. Over the next 13+ years Jose would go on to have a total of 4 heart attacks before he would have the first autologous myoblast stem cell transplant in the US. "They told me at the hospital that I had limited blood flow to the heart and they placed the first stent in one of my arteries. I might tell you there would be many more stents in my future." I asked, "During that first attack were you having any of the typical pains?" "No," said Jose, "I did not experience the pain in the shoulder or jaw or anywhere else as I have heard other people describing their event had. Come to think of it, I didn't have the typical pain during the last three heart attacks either."

THE SECOND HEART ATTACK: "It hit me about a year and half after the first one while I was sleeping. I awoke and felt like I needed to take a shower. This was a very cold night but there I am taking a shower with the windows open. I guess I was feeling pretty warm. As I am getting out of the shower, I suddenly realized I was beginning to feel very much like I had felt during the first attack. I woke my wife up and called the ambulance."

THE THIRD AND FOURTH HEART ATTACKS: "Happened about 4 years after the second one. As I've said, this attack did not cause me a lot of pain either and had I not had the other experiences I probably wouldn't have felt a need to even go to the hospital, but you know what? I AM ON MY WAY. I was actually having my third heart attack. Later that night while in the hospital I had my fourth attack!"

I asked Jose, how they described his condition and prognosis? "They told me more of my heart was deteriorating, particularly in the lower end of the heart. They inserted more stents." "How many stents now, Jose?" "Actually at this point when I left the hospital I had 9 stents working for me but as a couple of years ago the number increased to a total of 11 stents!" "Eleven stents? I wouldn't want to be standing behind you in line as you go through airport security."

"I continued working. I had a family depending on me, the guys I worked with understood I just couldn't sit home. They looked after me and didn't let me do the heavy work."

What is particularly amazing about Jose's case is that even with his low ejection fraction and numerous infarcts (attacks) continuing each time to destroy more and more of his heart, he still had not experienced the typical fatigue that a doctor would expect. Jose continues working and in spite of four heart attacks has still been able to go 11 minutes on a treadmill, reaching maximum output! I ask Jose, "So how do you become an early subject of myoblast stem cell transplant? How do you meet Dr. Sherman?

"At a given point around late 2002-2003 I have decided I am willing to try anything new out there that might help me. I tell my cardiologist that I am willing to be a guinea pig if necessary. He explains there have been studies going on in Europe and a Dr. Sherman would be beginning similar studies here in New York at the Mt. Sinai Medical Center. Long story short, it comes back that I am one of the first on the list. Now I keep calling and pushing to get into the program." As Jose explained to Dr. Sherman, "you guys are trying to do something to help keep me around a lot longer and I am grateful. Hopefully, others are going to benefit as well. Finally, the call came. 'We are ready for you.' I went to meet with Dr. Sherman and let me tell you, this guy is great! His attitude and concern made me feel very comfortable. This is one of the guys you want to hang out with, believe me. My family grew to love the guy also. As far as I know I was the first patient in the states. I am sure he was somewhat nervous, considering that he hadn't known me and he was taking on a new experimental technology. I told him, I'm here, so let's just do it! Dr. Sherman leveled with me, told me what had gone well and not so well with the initial studies. He would install a defibrillator as a safeguard in case something unforeseen went wrong. I told him hey, don't worry about it. I had no problem with having it installed as long as it was part of the study and I didn't have to pay for it. I looked at the procedure as something that needed to be done and I wanted to do it. It took several months of healing time after the defibrillator was installed before the team was ready to begin the stem cell procedures."

MEET MARCO ZELEDON: In 1998 Marco was 65 and living with his wife and family in Nicaragua. One day while he was searching for something in his closet, where of all places, he was struck with a heart attack. Today 8 years later and now age 73, he shares his journey of recovery, "I must have lost consciousness because my wife found me there on the floor about an hour and half later. I was taken to a hospital whose equipment and facility was very limited. They told me I had had an acute heart attack." Did they indicate the extent of the damage? "Well, I did overhear them say, we cannot move him today because if we do, he dies." In spite of this negative news, better news was coming for Marco. Fortunately, his nephew just happened to be a cardiologist and even more fortunate, his nephew was a visitor in Nicaragua at that very same time as Marco's attack. Dr. Christian Machado was vacationing at a beach resort when Marco had his attack. "Immediately upon hearing the news he came to the hospital and took control of my situation," explains Marco. "Things then moved quickly and the next day a medivac airplane equipped for cardiovascular care arrived from Florida. My nephew flew with me to the Providence Hospital in Southfield, Michigan where he practiced. I was put in ICU and remained there for 11 days." Marco, that is a long time in ICU—there must have been serious damage? Marco replies, "They had me on life saving machines for the first few days. I was later told they had to take heroic measures in many steps along the way in my care just to keep me alive. It was touch and go. They told me my ejection fraction was in the mid 20's and I was definitely in congestive heart failure. I had very little stamina. As I left the hospital I was told to take it easy and to not lift anything more than 25 lbs. It took about three months before I would start to feel stronger. I was active but very constrained in my activities. Anyhow, this was in 1998 and I have been doing pretty well since. Sometimes the water in my body would build up and I would go to the hospital and have it drained. I have been seeing my doctor Margolis here in Miami every 3 or 4 months. [James Margolis, M.D. is Director of Cardiovascular Research and Education at Miami International Cardiology Consultants.] I continued to eat "intelligently" as my doctor likes to call it and I have been taking my medications for the past 7 years since the attack."

Time for a Miracle

So Marco, how did you get the opportunity for the cell transplant? "This last year I began to really tire more easily. It became very obvious to my family that I was noticeably slowing down. Dr. Margolis had been looking into the information coming from Holland on the myoblast stem cell procedure. I believe that was around 2002. I was interested, but this process would require me (if I were accepted), to make many trips overseas for follow-up tests and evaluations. The money was one factor but the main reason was I didn't feel I would have the strength to go through the whole process. Dr. Margolis was concerned about me and the fact that we might be running out of time. He continued to believe getting the stem cells might be a very good situation for me. He approached Dr. Warren Sherman at one of the stem cell conferences and told him about me. An appointment was made and I visited Dr. Sherman in New York for a pre-evaluation. It was just this last October (4 months ago) that my doctor, my wife, and son all decided to go with me a second time to meet with Dr. Sherman. We all felt very comfortable with him and he believed I would be a good candidate for the procedure."

Marco continues, "The decision was made! I would have the stem cells taken from my own body and transplanted into my heart. In the beginning of November 2005 they withdrew the cells from my leg muscle to be cultured. I would be getting the higher dose of cells in contrast to the lower doses patients received in the first arm of the study. "On the 5th of December they decided they would inject the cells through 18 injections. One thing that was different in my case was not only how quickly the cells were reproduced but the very high number of cells that were cultured from my own cells." I explained to Marco that Bioheart's Chief of Staff, Scott Bromley, had assured me that their new laboratory in Sunrise Florida had new advanced procedures and technology in place to rapidly increase the number of cells and with a much shorter time to delivery. As a matter of fact added Marco, Bioheart's CEO Mr. Leonhardt flew to New York to be there personally to make sure everything was all right for me. I was able to watch the entire procedure on the monitor. It was a very interesting experience.

Sharing the Hope

A lot of readers who might want to explore the possibilities of becoming involved with one of the trials would like to know more about your experience and how much you have improved. As I hear you now Marco, your voice sounds very energetic and vital, are you aware of the difference? "If you had spoken to me before the operation you would have been aware you were talking to a very tired slow talking person. I would have been short of breath and it would require an effort for me to even talk."

Would you give me an idea for comparison as to how far you could have walked, say, six months before you received the cells and how far you can walk now after having the transplant? "Using the treadmill here where I am staying since my transplant, I walk .75 miles in 15 minutes. I guess that would mean three quarters of a mile." Ok, how far do you think you could have walked before New York? "I don't feel qualified to compare it in percentages, but this much I can tell you. Before receiving the cells I could walk maybe a half block and would be exhausted. I would be out of breath and have to stop. I had no energy. Today I feel very very good, like a new man, although I must say I have not seen my recent test results." The results must have been good or Dr. Sherman would not have released you to go to your home in Nicaragua? "Well he did say he doesn't need to see me again until June. But I myself feel like a new man. I swim and do my laps here in the pool, the other day I actually did short laps for an hour and I am pacing myself very well." Congratulations, Marco, send me a card when you get home!

The Road to Recovery

The prospects of early demise following a heart attack for both men and women are very real, but particularly among female patients. Fortunately, there has been a concerted effort by the American Heart Association and celebrity spokeswomen in bringing women to a greater awareness and need for more involvement with their own healthcare. It is after all the women who have been saving the lives of the men for the past 40-50 years. It has been the women who have taken the time to read the health articles and women who have encouraged their men to keep appointments for annual physicals and treadmills, adopt better eating habits and engage more frequently in some form of exercise. In contrast, women's cardiovascular heath care has not been a priority. A need for better education and preventive diagnostics for the female patient was very well supported in a study published in journal *Geriatrics and Gynecology*. The study had found their physicians had missed 34% of all heart attacks that occurred among women. Another discouraging statistic that supports a greater need for better diagnostics and preventive care for women is found in the comparison, 44% of women do not survive a full year following their first heart attack compared to 27% of men. The stakes are high and changes in lifestyle, eating habits, stress management and exercise routine must be made. Seventy-one percent of women do not survive the first year following their attack. Depression, too, often visits the heart attack victim and doctors recognize that it can be a very real complication of recovery.

CHAPTER 8

When It's All on the Line

Doctors are frequently forced to make difficult decisions in order to save a life. The following two situations demonstrate how different attending medical teams each reacted when faced with unique challenges. Constantly aware of their oath to "Do No Harm", physicians must weigh what the end result may be for a particular patient, when prescribing minimal treatment, staying within safe confines of the system may actually be contrary to the objective 'do no harm.' Most physicians gratefully will never be confronted with having to make such a decision, but for those rare and dire situations where the answer to save a life might lie outside the safe zone–what should the physician do? A doctor or team of doctors whose professional wisdom dictates they take the road less traveled–to save their patient may do so at some personal challenge to career and reputation. One of the cases I was referring to was an event that had captured worldwide attention two years earlier in which 16 year old Dimitri Bonneville, shot in the heart with a carpenter's nail gun, lay in ICU between life and death. The nail gun fired by a friend had lodged a large 3" nail directly into Dimitri's heart, resulting in a major heart attack. The second example, similar in consequence but remote in time, happened to a famous opera singer many decades earlier. In the one case a team quickly assembled at Beaumont Hospital in Michigan to evaluate and render assistance to the young man who laid in intensive care. Would the physicians brave a new frontier in performing a relatively unproven procedure that might give the young patient the best chance of recovery? The attending doctors in Michigan confronted with a decision in the young patient's case decided to do whatever necessary to save their young patient.

To learn more about what lead up to their decision to move forward, I needed to speak with Dr. Steven Timmis the young man's cardiologist associated with the Michigan hospital. I began the interview by asking the doctor what was the actual diagnosis and projected prognosis for the young patient, how serious was his condition following the nail gun incident? Dr. Timmis replied, "It was confirmed that Dimitri's artery had been literally shut down resulting in a major heart attack causing his ejection fraction to drop to a low 25%. As a young man of 25 years, the indications were that his heart had sustained a very significant degree of damage. There was complete loss of heart muscle in the heart region where the nail had penetrated." Additionally, the doctor explains, when Q waves on an EKG are deep, accompanied with persistent ST elevation, the combination suggests to the physician that the associated region of heart muscle is not going to recover." What then I asked, was involved in making the final decision to proceed?

Dr. Timmis explains, "After careful consultation involving the surgical staff, cardiologists and management—a decision was made to intervene to save the boy's life. The doctors would perform an experimental procedure based on a technology still in the experimental stage but that had previously been done in Europe. The doctors at Beaumont were not new to this science and technology having been studying heart stem cell transplantation for some time and were awaiting approval for a government grant to continue their studies. Much concerted effort had been invested according to Dr. Timmis, in preparation for this new therapy. The decision that was made, by current standards would be considered very advanced and somewhat, "outside the box." The procedure Dr. Timmis discussed would use the boy's own stem cells injected into the damaged areas of his heart. What was the consensus opinion of the team in moving forward? Dr. Timmis, "The general feeling was that this patient was doing very poorly and his condition was tenuous. We were able to stabilize him but his blood pressure remained very low and it would be a good while before we could take him off the ventilator. The one thing that was clear to the team was that the degree of injury was extensive. It was a high left ventricle anterior descending occlusion (LAD) involving a large area of the anterior wall including the apex. We knew the degree of reduction in heart function would be particularly severe."

So other options were considered? "Yes replied Dr. Timmis, and the assembled team considered both the short term and long term possibilities in their decision. We decided that the long-term outlook was particularly bleak. We performed both PET [positron emission tomography and Hi sensitivity MRI (magnetic resonance imaging) with contrast to further assess the damage helping to determine our course of action. Both of the technologies showed absolutely no viability in the areas damaged. The patients' EKG also confirmed a complete loss of viability."

You are about to perform a unique stem cell transplantation, using the boy's own heart stem cells. Had this particular procedure ever been done? "Yes, they had done a very similar successful transplant in Germany. We would remove cells from the patient's heart; culture them until we would have about 1,000,000 cells for each injection. We would do 5 injections totaling 5 million cells. We decided we would not be planting these cells in the heart itself as some programs are doing, but would plant the cells down along the side of the damaged ventricle. After cell transplantation the EF increased from 25% to 35% and over time became a significant 40%." Did the decision to break from the norm in applying this technology save this young man's life? Answering my own question, it apparently did, and therefore ultimately must have been the right call. However not everyone agreed. The hospital was denied its right to receive the grant it had previously applied for to become an integral part of stem cell research and application.

So What Does an Opera Singer's Death Have to do with the Beaumont Hospital?

At a given point in my conversation with Dr. Timmis, I wanted to share a true story that had happened in the life of the world's greatest opera singer, Enrico Caruso, as he lay on his deathbed in Sorrento, Italy. Enrico's wife, Dorothy, had taken him there to recuperate from complications from pleurisy that had turned to pneumonia, further complicated by the formation of an abscess, that was now draining into the singer's pleural cavity. As she later recounted in her memoirs, her husband's screams of pain throughout the night sounded like that of a tortured animal. Eight of Europe's finest physicians including the Bastinelli brothers [considered Rome's finest] were assembled to render care to Caruso whose death was now appearing inevitable. Enrico's wife had begged them to try something out of the ordinary, if necessary, to at least lance and drain the abscess, as had been done earlier in America. Clearly her husband's condition was already deemed terminal. As she would recount years later in her book, *Enrico Caruso, His Life and Death*, "I begged them to at least give my husband morphine and I finally had to inject the syringe myself. A transfusion? They agreed to only give him oxygen." As she would much later share on an interview, these men valued their reputations more than her husband's life. They were concerned that if the beloved Caruso died at their hands their reputations would be ruined— they chose to standby and watch the great tenor die rather than risk failing and damaging their careers.

Dimitri Bonneville and Enrico Caruso were two patients living many decades apart. At first glance they would certainly appear to have absolutely nothing at all in common, except both patients would require their physicians to take ultimate interventional steps to save their lives. One team of doctors did not, but thankfully, Dimmitri's team at Beaumont hospital did accept the challenge and rose to the occasion.

- The invention of the nail gun was an advanced piece of technology that has been welcomed by the building industry. It is reported that more than 250 (many fatal) accidents have occurred from nail gun use. The most recent case was reported in the national press in April 2006 in which a man had 26 nails removed from his skull and lived!

CHAPTER 9

University of Pittsburgh
Stem Cell Program

D r. Amit Patel is the Director of the Center for Cardiac Therapy at UPMC and Director of Cardiac Stem Cell Therapy at the McGowan Institute of Regenerative Medicine. Dr. Patel is the principal investigator of the only FDA surgically approved study using stem cells to strengthen the failing hearts of congestive heart failure patients. "The declining health of these patients waiting for a heart transplant, explained Dr. Patel, is so grave that an LVAD (left ventricle assist device) has to be implanted to literally keep them alive until a donor heart can be found." Dr. Patel in petitioning the FDA for approval to begin a trial, believed that if the agency would permit him and his team to inject the patients own stem cells directly into their failing hearts at the very same time as the LVAD device would be installed, the patient might experience an amazing unprecedented recovery. Dr. Patel explained, "In effect, as part of our proof of concept we were saying, 'Look, the cells we have implanted in patients overseas are now at the very least proving the technology and science to be safe, showing definite early patient benefit. That benefit and the groundwork already established should be sufficient to justify our getting started with similar therapies here in the states." Additional factors for consideration helped move Dr. Patel's petitions forward. For instance, his having done 200 similar procedures in Argentina, Uruguay, Thailand and with limited work in Italy, Greece and Ecuador would be considered in the equation. He explained, these patients who did so well did not receive any device or assistance from outside their own bodies.

- They did not receive stents.

- They did not receive bypass.

- They were not given any other procedures.

All they were given was bone marrow or blood-derived cells, extracted from their own bone marrow or blood.

The FDA Approves Two Applications

The FDA granted permission to begin not one trial but two.

1. LVAD plus Cells (patient's own marrow cells along with a device.)

2. Bypass surgery plus cells. (Open heart surgery and stem cells simultaneously).

During our interview, Dr. Patel explained what he hoped to see accomplished in the studies; "When the implanted device would be removed in anticipation of the actual heart transplant, we would be looking at a native heart that presumably, already would have had 5 to 6 months on the artificial LVAD device. Besides the benefit of having the life-extending device in place, they would also have the additional strength of their own stem cells that had been injected 5 or 6 months earlier. As the doctor explained, "If our theory and approach were correct, what you would then have would be a patient with a newly rejuvenated heart that in all probability would not need the transplant at all!" Everything to gain. In effect, another miracle would have taken place and hope for thousands desperately waiting for an available heart match to become available would have another less involved and dramatic option. Additionally there should not have been additional risk for the patient. Another very real consideration is that heart transplants have very poor survival rates after five six and seven years plus they require the patient to be on a lifetime of immune suppressant drugs.

The early results of the ongoing trial under Dr. Patel's direction reported in the December 2005 (*Journal of Thoracic and Cardiovascular Surgery*): ten of the study patients were given bypass and ten received both bypass and bone marrow cells at the same time. As the early results would confirm, the patients who received the transplant and the bypass together did much better than those who were only given the stem cells.

Proving the Technology

In 1992, Dr. Patel began working with small clinics in Argentina who were performing standard bypass surgeries. As he explained, "There were patients whom we felt could not be successful coronary bypass grafting candidates. However, if they still had live viable heart muscle, we would do stem cell bone marrow derived implantation. We actually harvested the cells from the patient's own hip-bones and put them into the heart muscle using purified filtered bone marrow."

(Continues page 154)

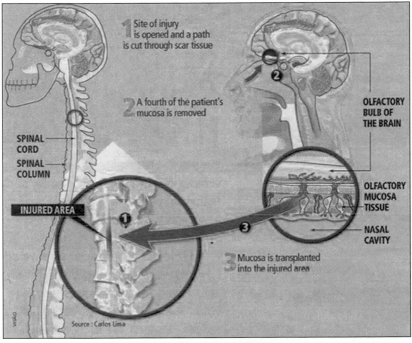

Fig. 8 Spinal injury repair.

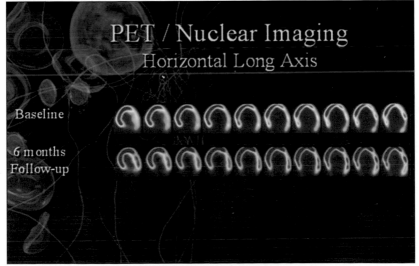

Fig. 9 Dr. Cohen MRI before and after results.
The bottom line of MRI images shows increased viable heart function.

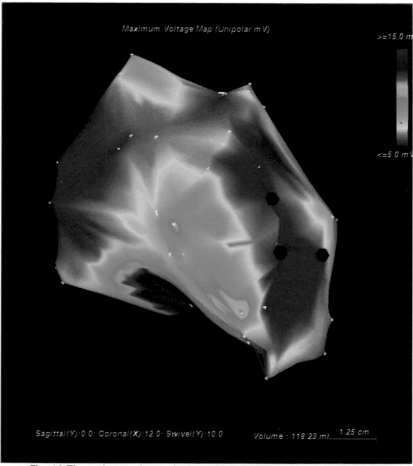

Fig. 10 The red area shows destroyed heart muscle from previous heart attack—the green/yellow areas denote healthy tissue. The 3 black spots indicate where Duane's own stem cells were injected into his damaged heart.

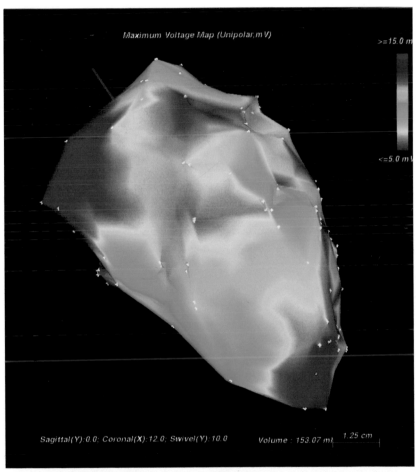

Fig. 11 At 3 month follow-up using 3-dimensional Noga Mapping, the previous dead heart muscle (red) is shown replaced with viable healthy (green/yellow) heart tissue and repair will continue over time. Images appear by special permission. Before and after scanning performed with Cordis Noga Mapping.

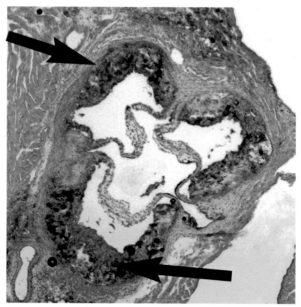

Fig. 12 Dark area denotes advanced plaque in an older mouse artery
before VPC treatment.

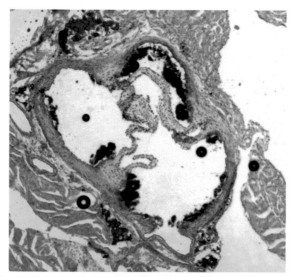

Fig. 13 Note: Plaque is almost totally dissolved after treatment
with VPC cells from a young healthy mouse.

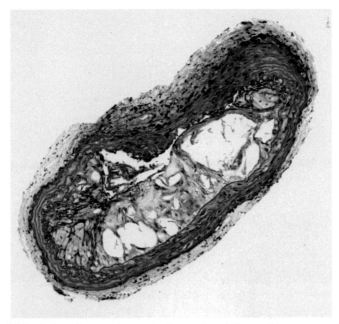

Fig. 14 Dark ring shows advanced atherosclerosis in an older mouse artery.

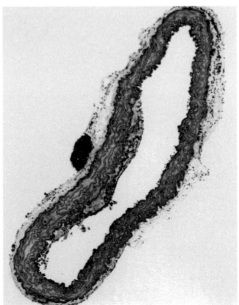

Fig. 15 After VPC treatment, with cells from a young mouse
plaque is significantly reduced.

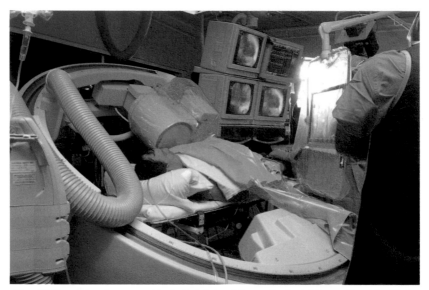

Fig. 16 Preparing for a myoblast skeletal cell transplant at Arizona Heart Institute.

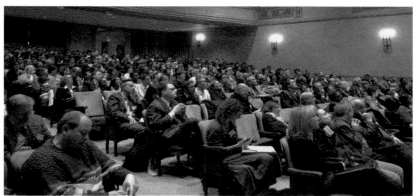

Fig. 17 Columbia University's 2nd annual International Stem Cell Conference,
American Academy of Medicine,New York City,
courtesy of the Cardiovascular Research Foundation.

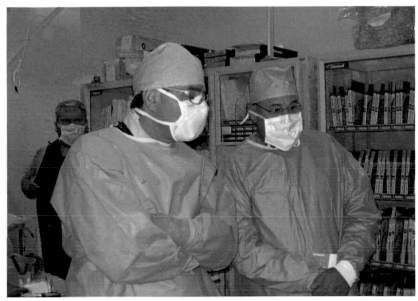

Fig. 18 Dr. Dib (left) explains the capabilities of Noga Mapping to the author.

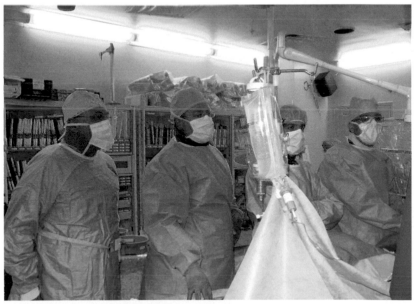

Fig. 19 Author (far left) observes Dr. Dib and team members performing a cell transplant on an 82 year old patient.

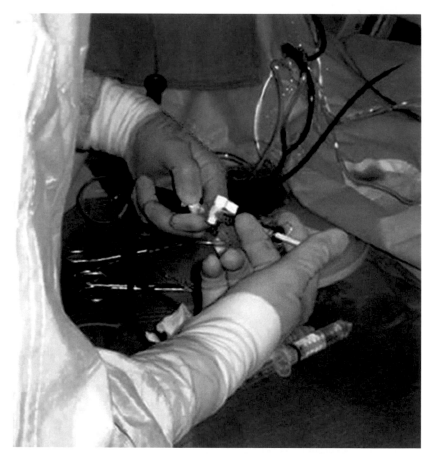

Fig. 20 Loading the catheter for intracoronary injection.

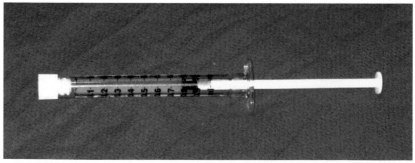

Fig. 21 Myogen's syringe with 1,000,000 cells prepared for transplant.

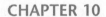

CHAPTER 10

Congestive Heart Failure, ᵃⁿEpidemic

*W*ith more than 22 million current cases of congestive heart failure worldwide and 5 million in this
country alone augmented by a growing number of 450-
500,000 each year, heart failure is a failing health prob-

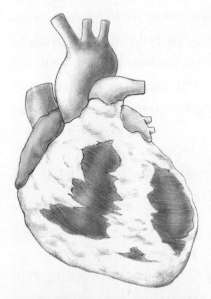

Fig. 22 A healthy normal sized heart.
Illustrated by Jeeyoung.

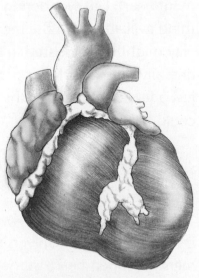

Fig. 23 A severely enlarged heart
in advanced failure.
Illustrated by Jeeyoung.

lem. Many of these patients are currently waiting and hoping against hope that a matching donor heart will become available in time to save them. Unfortunately, with the great and growing number of heart failure patients in the national registry, not everyone will receive help in time. When a congestive heart failure patient becomes advanced in their disease, the progression leads to an escalated loss in quality of life and eventual premature death. According to Dr. Patel, these ischemic patients qualify as heart failure patients with an ejection fraction of 35% or less, [normal being 55-65%.]

Families and physicians ever since heart transplant surgery was invented have been left frustrated and bewildered over their unfulfilled hope of receiving a replacement heart. Left wondering why there hadn't been something available from the medical community that in some way might have assisted in keeping their patient or loved one alive just a little longer? Was that too much to ask, just a few weeks or months until a qualifying donor heart could have been found?

The LVAD, Left Ventricle Assist Device to the Rescue

Apparently, world-renowned heart surgeon Dr. Michael DeBakey of Baylor University, a pioneer in the development of open-heart surgery was also wondering. Dr. DeBakey along with David Saucier of NASA's Johnson Space Center would in 1995 develop the first life extending LVAD device and bring hope to hundreds of thousands. Their original device could now maintain patient heart stability for up to a full year if necessary. A newer improved model has shown, during the manufacturer's phase two studies, to even provide longer patient survival time and improvement in quality of life.

Michael Debakey's LVAD Answered the First Question

Dr. Patel is attempting to answer the second question in bringing an alternative solution to heart failure and a need for heart transplantation by repairing the damaged failing heart using bone marrow derived adult stem cells.

Pioneering the Effort Forward, the First Case

Juan Neumann of Uruguay, in March, 2004, became the first non-open heart stem cell implant case done in not only South America but anywhere in the world. Juan had not had a heart attack, but did have very significant, sub-normal heart function of 17%. He details his story for me, "About seven years earlier doctors had found that my heart was not working very well, they checked my arteries and decided they were all ok." Juan's case would be one of idiopathic non-ischemic cardiomyopathy. I asked Juan if he could recall having contracted any infections as a young man that might have contributed to his current condition? "When I was six years old growing up," replied Juan, "living in La Paz, Bolivia, I had a serious case of pneumonia and two years later came down with a life threatening case of Typhus. La Paz is about 4,000 meters elevation and my doctors told me the clean air in my recovery had been good for my lungs." As Juan explained, since he was a boy he had always been active and involved with exercise, which he believed had served him well since his childhood illness. In spite of his low heart function in 2004 at the time of his transplant, he had still been able to continue working. "My doctor had been able to increase my heart output with medication and workouts at the gym." During this period of time Juan was overdue to have a colon operation, which had been postponed earlier because of his health. "My doctor thought it would not be good for me at the time to undergo a strenuous surgery. He believed however, that if I could improve my heart function up to 30% with medications and regular exercise at the gym, they could then proceed. When I went to see my cardiologist, Dr. Robert Pagannini, he said Juan, I think I have some very encouraging news for you." He told me about some exciting things that were being done with stem cells for heart failure and that an American doctor was here to teach him the new surgery. This would be the first time the procedure would be done in South America. Even though I did not know much about stem cells, I immediately said "yes, I would like to take advantage of this surgery."

Juan would later learn that his was also the first stem cell, non-open heart surgery done for heart failure in not only South America, but also anywhere else in the world. Juan explained, "They removed bone marrow from my hip, and made 3 very tiny incisions beneath my left arm. The area was, I would say about two inches." To put this in a timeframe, it took place in March 2004 and Dr. Patel and the doctors in Uruguay now have had the benefit of a full two year follow-up to evaluate the continued success of Juan's procedure. Here is proof of the benefit. The success of Juan's surgery was already evident two weeks following the cell implant. His ejection fraction rose from 30% prior to surgery to a new high of 45% and today Juan's current readings two years out have maintained according to the echocardiogram at a significant 46%! Juan recalled the number of cells extracted from the bone marrow in his hip to his heart to be 42M.

Ischemic Cardiomyopathy and Non-Ischemic Cardiomyopathy

Dr. Patel explained, "100% of the heart stem cell studies currently going on in the country are dealing with the two different cardiovascular areas, one is idiopathic cardiomyopathy, the other is ischemic coronary disease. Forty percent of patients who present with non-ischemic disease have a weakened heart but they do not necessarily have blockages in their arteries. Hawaiian singer Don Ho of *Tiny Bubbles* fame was an example of one with idiopathic cardiomyopathy heart failure and had an incredibly low ejection fraction of 10%. He had been told his heart was basically destroyed and given no hope for recovery. Dr. Patel implanted the singer's own stem cells in his heart in a procedure done in Thailand in December of 2005. Less than two months later, the singer was again performing strenuous 90-minute shows (although not as many) as he had years earlier. He is another living miracle. There is a distinct difference in what constitutes ischemic cardiomyopathy and what constitutes a classification of non-ischemic cardiomyopathy. Quite simply, the first type is the result of the common risk factors we have heard about for the past 50 years. Smoking, high cholesterol, high fat intake, stress, sedentary life style and poor dietary habits. The other form, non-ischemic, may have resulted from chronic uncontrolled high blood pressure or perhaps a previous viral or bacterial infection affecting the heart. There are also unknown causes that result in a diagnosis of non-ischemic disease.

According to Dr. Patel, both classifications of patients qualify for a heart failure diagnosis if the ejection fraction is 35% or lower. Dr. Patel explains there are many ongoing trials concentrating on bringing hope to the 60% of heart failure patients with ischemic heart failure. So, if coronary heart disease would explain the 60% of the 5 million cases who have entered this classification, what about the remaining percentage of patients? The question Dr. Patel is attempting to answer, is what help can be offered the other 40%?

A Case of Non-Ischemic Cardiomyopathy

By age 17, Jeannine was becoming aware that she had something in heart dysfunction when during a routine physical her high school nurse informed her that she was displaying an irregular heartbeat. It would be about six months later that Jeannine, upon seeing her regular family doctor, would bring the nurse's comment to his attention. He examined her, ordered some tests and called a few days later to say that his diagnosis for her condition was cardiomyopathy. Jeannine was not symptomatic at that time and shared that in the early years following the diagnosis everything still seemed quite normal. During her 20's she described herself as the typical twenty year old. "Working full time, I went out with my friends dancing on the weekends and at certain times I worked two jobs." Her disease was not at that time hampering her activities, nor was she aware of it affecting her energy level. As time went on Jeannine recalled that she was prone to tire more easily.

"I thought, perhaps the drop in energy might be that I was just getting a little older. Perhaps I had picked up a couple of pounds or I could blame it on a lack of exercise." During this period of time Jeannine said she met her husband to be and was concerned if the relationship would culminate in marriage, "Would I be able to carry a child or would I have to disappoint my husband by informing him after the fact, that I had been earlier advised by a physician not to become pregnant?" Being a conscientious individual she explained during our interview that she went to see a cardiologist for his evaluation and advice. Looking at her ejection fraction, which had fluctuated between 25-30, the doctor's determination was that she was good to go. "I was told," said Jeannine, "carrying a child should not be a problem as long as I was closely monitored." It wasn't long after that meeting that Jeannine's disease was taking a more serious turn. As she explained, "I was working a full week, maintaining a home and doing the house work. I was becoming exhausted. My husband and I made two decisions. One that I would quit work to be a full time homemaker and two, that we would have our first child. After about the third month of my pregnancy I began having chest pains. I visited my family doctor who informed me that I was displaying arrhythmias and I should see a cardiologist ASAP." Jeannine had earlier encountered difficulty with a doctor who did not take her symptoms seriously, thinking she was too young and healthy looking to be seriously ill. The next time Jeannine would go to an appointment with a new doctor she would take her mother-in-law with her for support. As she shared, "This time in meeting the new doctor my apprehension was not warranted. He immediately determined that my condition was indeed very serious. He explained he would do what he could to get me through this pregnancy but felt compelled to tell me— that if it became a condition that put my life in great jeopardy, he would have to terminate the pregnancy to save my life."

By the 27th week Jeannine recalls having difficulty breathing and when she met with her OBGYN the response she got was, "who said you were allowed to get pregnant?" I explained said Jeannine, "I had sought a cardiologist's opinion prior to conceiving. His concern was that my baby was not going to receive the proper amount of oxygen because I was myself now becoming deficient. To help the baby's lung development the doctor injected me with steroids, when they admitted me to the hospital they found a blood clot had formed in my heart. From 27 weeks forward I self injected blood anticoagulants and during week 33 I again went back into the hospital, this time with premature contractions." Two weeks later Jeannine's water broke and she gave birth at 35 weeks to her 5 lb 4 oz baby boy. Sometime later, she added she saw her cardiologist who performed an echocardiogram. "A few days later the doctor called me to say the results of the echo were lower than before." In spite of trying different medications which seemed to bring a short term result, I never got back to feeling as well as I had before the pregnancy. My symptoms were shortness of breath, palpitations and for the first time my feet and ankles were beginning to retain water. It had become apparent that the pregnancy was what finally put me over the edge in regard to my cardiomyopathy. Money was short and I decided to take some kind of job to help the situation. I wanted to feel better about myself I thought the ideal job would be to work in daycare about four hours a day. As a fringe benefit, I would be able to also watch over my two year old." Any of you who know how much energy is sucked out of you while chasing around a group of kindergarten kids or even your own kids would understand how totally exhausting this type employment would be for someone with stamina issues. Jeannine was at this time experiencing high blood pressure and palpitations accompanied by dizzy spells. She continued, "Finally after about 3 weeks I had to stop working. I was so devastated with this inability to function and take care of my boy that it sent me into a very pronounced depressive state." Jeannine had come to the realization that she had a severe illness that was not going to get better. She had done her homework and knew that at any time she was at high risk for sudden cardiac death. As she explained, "I began putting my will together, detailing my wishes for my son, taking care of the insurance and all the details including my internment. I can't imagine how it must have felt for my husband having to go through all of this but that is how final it all looked to me and I just wanted to have everything in order."

What makes this such an encouraging story is when Jeannine was at her lowest ebb, a miracle was about to happen! In her desperate search for any answer in 2005 she remembered that she had read a brief paragraph about stem cells for the heart and (according to the article) researchers were looking into treating heart failure with stem cells. "While I was at my brother's house doing my taxes I went online and searched. I filled out the medical questioner online form and submitted it to a company called Vescell." One problem, the information was that they treated ischemic heart failure and Jeannine's case was diagnosed as being non-ischemic heart failure. Jeannine was excited as she relayed the following scenario to me, "About five months later I received a phone call from overseas. At first I thought it was a telemarketer because he referring to a survey I had filled out. Suddenly the discussion changed to the subject of heart failure. He explained his company had a procedure that may be able to help me and asked if I would be interested in following up? To begin with, the logistics would require me to fly to Thailand to have the procedure and it would cost between 40-60K. It wasn't an issue of the hospital location" Jeannine said, "I would have gone to the moon if necessary, but money was certainly a major issue plus the fact that the procedure had not been FDA approved nor was it covered by insurance. These were all no-gos! The company representative was enthusiastic about a great new doctor they were working with from the University of Pittsburgh Medical Center, a Dr. Amit Patel." The representative mentioned that Dr. Patel had developed a procedure that could help her. "I was put in contact with Dr. Patel and with my own cardiologist to interpret and qualify the information we were receiving from Thailand. We were making sure everything was legitimate." Her doctor consulted with Dr. Patel whose credentials are outstanding and having met him myself at the Academy of Medicine in New York, I can say his manner is calm and confident. To make this come to pass there was an amazing amount of logistics to bring together, in a very short period of time. It was well into the month of May and Dr. Patel was already scheduled to be in Bangkok the last week in May to teach Thai surgeons the procedure. If Jeannine was to take advantage of this rare opportunity she would have to first travel to Pittsburgh to meet with Dr. Patel and undergo MRI and whatever other diagnostics would be required. Oh yes, one other small issue would be raising 40-60 K in a few days!

Here is another piece of this amazing timeline story. Jeannine received a phone call from the blood clinic in Israel on a Friday with the instruction that her blood must be drawn in the U.S. by the following Tuesday in order to be shipped to Israel to have her stem cells prepared and cultured for the procedure prior to her arrival in Thailand. Time obviously was an almost paralyzing factor that threatened to end this endeavor before Jeannine would get her chance for a miracle. The cells would arrive in Thailand May 25th the same day as Jeannine's proposed arrival. Jeannine recalled, "at this time I still did not have a ticket, but if something is really being guided and meant to happen, as apparently this case will prove, nothing is going to stop it! When I got to the university I explained that I hadn't worked in years and we were a young couple without assets raising our child, and there was no way we could afford the full amount. My husband and I figured we could come up with 15K at the most. We could mortgage our home and I could put enough on my credit card to buy the plane ticket. How great was it that the Israeli company agreed to donate the costs of my stem cell preparation and as if it was scripted, one by one the obstacles were going by the wayside–everything was working for me to have this procedure."

Jeannine explained how intent she was upon going for it! She said, "My mother had been praying for God to heal her daughter's heart," even though Jeannine had told her mother, "there is nothing the doctors can do for me! If you want to pray for something, pray for a heart transplant." Her mother responded with, "No I am praying for God to heal your heart!" Jeannine's mother and her husband were basically praying for a miracle. Jeannie was just praying for something good to happen. Suddenly the news came, "Dr. Patel was going to fix my heart, my mom was right. When I finally got ready to go for the operation, my mom put me on just about every prayer chain in the country and the week before I left, the elders of the church prayed over me." An interesting side note. Jeannine explained to me that although she had never before flown she approached this experimental journey with no doubts or reservations.

Post Surgery Results

"The surgery went as planned and I was checked out of the hospital following a medical evaluation. I was given my after care instructions a few days later and flew home.

When I arrived home, I remembered going to bed at 7:00 P.M. I awoke around 6:00 AM with so much new revived energy that I went outside and literally began weed whacking! It had been just about one week since the successful surgery in Bangkok. When I asked what differences she was experiencing she replied, "Prior to surgery I would sleep most of the day. Now since the surgery, I would only require one nap a day and the length of time I needed to rest became shorter and shorter with each passing week. Another pre-surgery symptom that had left was a previously frequent need to get up during the night for trips to the bathroom because of fluid retention. Significantly, during even my first and second week upon returning from Thailand, I was sleeping through each night and I would awaken completely rested. Prior symptoms were disappearing one by one until finally they were completely gone. Because the operation required entrance from my side directly into the heart, it had been necessary to deflate my lung. That soreness may have been the most lingering aspect until it, too, finally resolved." The very last side affect to leave was the swelling in her feet, which Jeannine was happy to say, "This too had completely left."

At the 3-month follow-up her ejection fraction was recorded at 41 up from 31 before treatment and dramatically up from 25 as it had been originally diagnosed when she was just 17 years old. Her heart failure rating went down from a severe class 3 to a class one and

Jeannine Lewis today has completed a very successful 6 month follow-up according to Dr. Patel. Thank you Jeannine for your inspiring story and the courage to go for it!

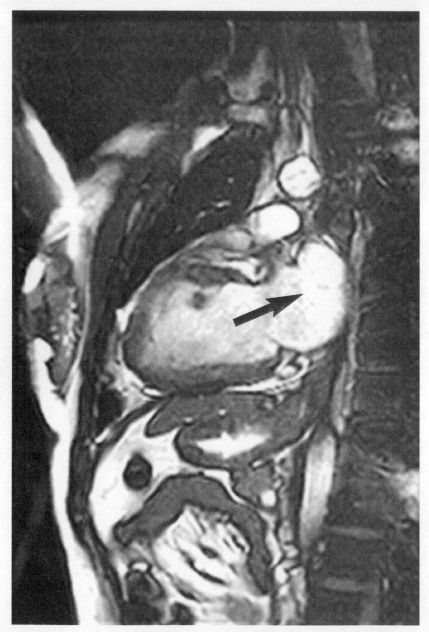

Fig. 24 MRI A heart enlarged 2 ½ times before stem cell treatment.
Shown by special permission.

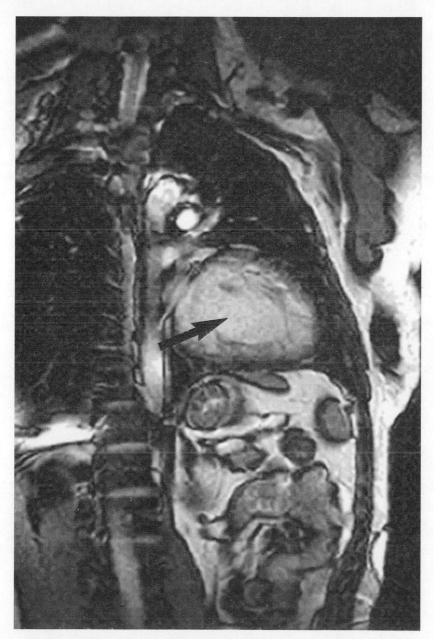

Fig. 25 MRI Shows the heart size (at 9 months follow-up) returned to normal.
Shown by special permission.

CHAPTER 11

Sleep Apnea and CHF

A ccording to Columbia University's Department of Otolaryngology, there are 20 million people positive for Obstructive Sleep Apnea Syndrome (OSAS) and another 5.4 million with OSAS who go undiagnosed. Sleep apnea can be a very serious, life-threatening ailment and should be acknowledged as such among heart disease patients and in particular among those with an arrhythmia, hypertension or heart failure diagnosis. What is the deciding determination for a diagnosis of OSAS? According to the university, when someone does not breathe for a ten second interval and this happens at least 5 times in an hour, the individual can assume he or she has some degree of apnea. The National Commission on Sleep Disorders estimates that 38,000 cardiovascular deaths caused by sleep apnea occur each year. Mayo Clinic cardiologist, Virend Somers, M.D., PhD., conducted a study that found more than twice as many cardiac deaths occur during sleeping compared to the waking hours. There are mixed reports concerning the number of people who expire in their sleep. It may actually be much higher than what is reported. There is a possible reason for the difficulty in determining the actual numbers. When someone dies during sleep from any cause, it is assumed they died of a heart attack and therefore sudden cardiac death. In fact the patient may have actually died as a direct cause of complications set in motion by one of two forms of sleep apnea, either central or obstructive.

An individual, depending on the severity of their ailment, can literally be awakened as many as 300 times a night. These individuals wake up tired, often falling asleep during their work hours or simply struggling through their day just to keep awake. According to the National Safety Council, the statistics on automobile fatalities due to sleep apnea number 15,000 deaths per year. The agency also claims that 800,000 related automobile accidents happen per year. A person must be sleeping uninterruptedly for several hours in order to enter the deepest most meaningful sleep. The person with apnea is awakened continually throughout the night and may never receive the quality sleep they require. It is very important for patients and doctors to understand the link between sleep apnea and heart failure as the connection is very often overlooked.

The Heart Failure/Apnea Connection

A study on adults entitled, *Sleep Apnea in 81 Ambulatory*

Male Patients With Stable Heart Failure by Javaheri, Liming and colleagues appeared in Circulation 1998. This study of sleep apnea and the result of repetitive asphyxia found that apnea has an adverse affect on the function of the heart. The patients recruited for the study had been diagnosed with heart failure and had been recorded with a mildly low left ventricle ejection output of 45%. Briefly, the study found that patients with this disorder have a high degree of atrial fibrillation and ventricular arrhythmias, both very serious life threatening disorders.

Sleep apnea is more than a minor annoyance; it can be a life-threatening ailment. The left ventricle becoming enlarged and weakened over time is often the cause of "sudden death." A wife can give her husband, or a husband his wife, a pretty good idea of the duration of episodes between breaths. God knows he or she isn't able to sleep anyway so he or she can pretty well monitor the intensity and frequency. Of course, women also snore, sleep apnea is not a gender based ailment. A study reported in the *American Journal of Epidemiology* in mid 2002, involving 70,000 nurses, claimed that women who snore release a hormone that creates a pathway to insulin resistance. That pathway can predispose them to type II diabetes. Now that the medical profession has corrected the misconception that heart disease is reserved for the male population, so must snoring and sleep apnea among women be addressed as a risk factor as well.

Being overweight is one of the most obvious reasons

for apnea. When one gains weight on the exterior of the neck and throat area, the weight is also gained internally within the back of the throat (pharynx) affecting the space between the tongue, the soft palate and pharynx. With time and added weight, the tissue on either side of the back of the throat can lose elasticity and encroach upon the air pathway. There are numerous snoring aids on the market. There are also surgeries. Allergies and swollen sinus membranes compromise one's ability to breath through their nose forcing open-mouth breathing, setting the apnea in motion. There is a condition called "positional apnea" created when the airway is choked by sleeping in a particular position. As an example, some individuals do not have a problem with central apnea but will consistently snore when they sleep on their back or on their side. Sleeping on one's stomach for some patients actually brings some relief of symptoms as well for some patients.

The true way of diagnosing this illness is to submit to a sleepover in a sleep deprivation-monitoring clinic. Here, under professional scrutiny, the patient's REM (rapid eye movement) vital signs, number of sleep interruptions and breathing episodes are monitored. This procedure can be expensive but many insurance companies do recognize this illness and most pay for the evaluation. The good news is that there is a 70% remedy rate for sleep apnea when one is diagnosed. The *Breathe Rite* nasal strips you see on NFL football players and other athletes actually bring a degree of relief for many snorers and might be considered the first line of defense before trying anything else. You don't have to be an NFL athlete to benefit from these little strips and amazingly; they can really provide serious benefit for many patients. In a good number of cases this breathing aid is all that is needed to keep the airway open, particularly if the problem resulted from sinus congestion or allergies. If you awaken in the morning with a dry mouth, you can pretty well deduce that you have been breathing through your mouth during the night and it may be a pretty good indication that you are a snorer whether or not you are experiencing apnea will need more evaluation.

CHAPTER 12

The Specially Tailored
Minneapolis Heart Institute Programs

D r. Timothy Henry is Director of all nine cardiovascular programs at the Minneapolis Heart Institute. Included among the nine are the stem cell trials. He could certainly have discussed the exciting results documented in the cell trials during our interview time together but was kind enough, at my request, to explain three very important subjects that had only been mentioned in passing earlier in the book. The three areas Dr. Henry focused his attention on were EECP® (external enhanced counterpulsation), the studies on prayer and the OPTIMIST program for the no option patient, a program of particular importance to Dr. Henry.

Dr. Timothy Henry on Alternative Programs

"We are looking at a group of patients with coronary artery disease who are not good candidates for either bypass or angioplasty. These patients," asserts Dr. Henry, "have basically been deemed 'No Option Patients,' having been told by their physicians there is nothing more that can be done for them. They are sent home. We decided at the Institute after much thought to use the name *Options In Myocardium Ischemic Syndrome Therapies*, which is how the name OPTIMIST was attached to the program. It certainly is a better choice of acronym than no option patient."

"To begin with, the standard method for determining a patient's qualification for the OPTIMIST program is the stress test." Dr. Henry continues with the criteria, "Eighty percent of the patients entering the program have already had the benefit of drugs like nitroglycerin, beta blockers and various other agents. These patients have all had the normally administered technologies and medications before they come to our program for evaluation. In spite of all that has been made available to them in care and therapy they are still failing and forty percent are also dealing with a diagnosis of diabetes. These patients are unfortunately in a very serious condition.

"I believe," says Dr. Henry, "we currently have the largest national database of about 1,200 patients nationwide who fit the criteria just outlined. What is very interesting about this group of patients is that they don't actually succumb in large numbers as one might think. They live quite long, but there is significant impairment to their quality of life. Anxiety, fear and depression are very real among these patients. In our information we find that these negative aspects are found almost entirely in 100% of this class of patient. Let me rephrase that last statement; one hundred percent are depressed but it is just that some have a greater degree of depression than others."

How does the clinic determine which program is right for a given patient? Dr. Henry answers, "Frequently, there are several approaches that might be helpful for an individual. However, because we have programs and sub-programs, one may be more beneficial than another for a particular patient." So you can tailor the program to fit the patient? "In a matter of speaking, yes, at the outset we have to determine first of all if theirs is a case that cannot be fixed by bypass or angioplasty: We start with 4 determining factors:

Risk factor modification

a. Establishing and controlling very low LDL.

b. Controlling patient blood pressure.

c. Prescribing anti-platelet medication.

d. Maximum medical management with beta blockers, ACE inhibitors or whatever is required to give them maximum benefit.

"As a comprehensive program we next look at what we have available for the patient by looking at some mundane but necessary criteria including logistics. As example," states Dr. Henry, "a patient would have great difficulty in traveling 6 hours over a 6 or 7 week period of time for EECP® treatments."

The Minneapolis Heart Institute has many programs and concentrates on responding to the specific need of a particular patient. If help can be found for those whose options are disappearing, the Minneapolis Heart Institute may be their best hope.

When They Have Given up on You, Where do You Turn for Help?

What happens when someone regrettably enters the classification of a NO-OPTION heart patient when every possible means of risk reduction, management and intervention has already been tried with minimal or limited result? What happens when a concerned physician must reluctantly throw in the towel, realizing there are no more magic potions and no more answers in his or her medical bag of tricks? There are thousands of such patients across the country that find themselves in this predicament everyday. Peter Pierce was such a patient. After a long battle with cardiovascular problems it would be the final prognosis from Peter's physician, Maria-Teresa P. Olivari, MD, FACC, that convinced him to seek the OPTIMIST program. Peter remembers, "My doctor, in the presence of my wife and kids, had honestly and candidly expressed her concern. She said very discreetly, this is about it. Meaning there wasn't much more they could do for me. There just wasn't any medical solution as I had explored all other possibilities—

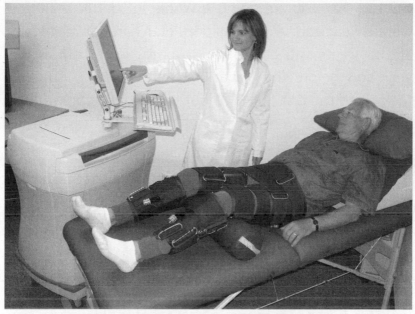

Fig. 26 ECP Photo. Courtesy of Cardiomedics.

none were left." ECP, EECP® is a methodology that literally forces the body to create small new collateral 'bypasses' around seriously blocked arteries and has been considered particularly beneficial for angina patients. Peter *did not* have angina but the procedure interestingly proved effective nonetheless.

Meet Peter

Good morning Peter, is this a good time to talk? "Yes it is, this is a fine time, I have about 45 minutes before I have to leave for my tee time." Peter is excited, because as he explains, he would be going out to play a full 18 holes of golf. I remarked, 18 holes, that tells me right off the bat that you are doing a whole lot better than you were a year ago. A year before Peter had completed 34 EECP® treatments at the Minneapolis Heart Institute. "A year ago before the treatments says Peter, "I couldn't make it to the first hole without being out of breath and fatigued, so yes from my way of measuring I am a whole lot better today."

I asked Mr. Pierce if he would not mind retracing his steps through his journey to his eventual appearance at the Heart Institute? "Well," replies Peter, "I'm 72 now and I was 68 years old when I had my first heart attack which incidentally was a week after my doctor, had given me a clean bill of health following my annual physical." Where have we heard that scenario before? Had they given you a stress test during that physical? "No, the doctor said I didn't need one. I had my heart attack in the fall of 1998 and in January of 1999 the following year, I had quadruple bypass surgery. I remained in the ICU for three days after the operation and while there, suffered a minor stroke. It took me a while to recover but I dealt with it and moved on. Since 1999, I have continued to see a cardiologist for follow-ups."

"A couple of years ago I noticed that I wasn't feeling particularly good and got to wondering if there just might be something else out there that could be done to help me? I was thinking perhaps a new remedy or some breakthrough in development, waiting for me right around the corner. A very good friend of mine, a retired surgeon, who incidentally also had experienced an earlier heart attack, suggested that I go over to the Minneapolis Heart Institute. I took his advice and met a Dr. Daniel who after checking me over suggested the possibility of my having a pacemaker installed. I believe my ejection fraction at that time was very low, at around 20. I followed up with a Dr. Olaveri whose specialty is congestive heart failure. Within a few days I was the proud owner of a new pacemaker." Peter explains at that time he was on a fair amount of medication and it was making him (as he said) very tired. Were you on a beta blocker I ask, because beta blockers slow the heart rate. "Yes, I had been on Coreg® and wanted off. One of the most common complaints of patients on this class of drug is the fatigue. "Now last summer I was really feeling exhausted, I had put on between 15-20 lbs in a relatively short period of time. I am sure the added weight contributed to my constant tiredness and on three occasions during that period, I ended up in the ER. The third time I was actually admitted to the hospital and remained there for a week. Fortunately my own personal doctor, Dr. Olaveri, was the doctor on duty for that entire week. It turned out to be a blessing because there were three important issues that she addressed for me during my stay: I was put on a low sodium diet after learning that a lot of the weight I had gained was water weight, which they proceeded to eliminate with diuretics. At this point Dr. Olaveri discussed the possibility of my getting EECP® treatments."

"EECP® was something I had read about earlier in the Minneapolis Heart Institutes' Foundation newsletter. My doctor explained that even though the treatments are normally prescribed for someone with angina (which I did not have) she said we could take a look at it to see if it might indeed help my shortness of breath and loss of energy. She referred me to Anil K. Poulose, MD, FACC, who worked with Dr. Henry in the research area. I was given some preliminary tests, scans etc and was told 'OK, let's give it a whirl!'

Pete how would you describe your condition at this point? How did you feel overall? "I would describe it that I was like a vegetable as I could hardly do anything. I even had a real tough time walking. As an example, if I walked a hundred yards I would have to stop and catch my breath along the way—as far as my energy level was concerned I literally had none. Basically, it had become difficult for me to do just about any function at all and to be honest, I felt so lousy I don't mind telling you I had gotten to the point where I didn't really care what happened. That was until I would realize what my illness was doing to my wife and family. That should give you a pretty good idea of how I felt both physically and emotionally. Anyway, my retired friend, the former surgeon I told you about, went with me to Minneapolis Heart to try and learn if there were any options for me. The doctor we met with mentioned the ongoing programs with stem cells. Basically there were three possibilities for me: Stem cell therapy (adult stem cells), gene therapy (angiogenesis—to create new blood vessels) and EECP® (to develop collateral arteries)."

"I decided along with my surgeon friend that we should begin with EECP®. The worst that would happen is that I would have invested 35 one hour sessions of my time." The 35 treatments can be done two at a time which shortens the duration of the therapy to 17 days." Peter decided on the doubled up option but in a few days felt extremely tired and decided along with his advisors to modify the schedule and limit the therapy to one-hour sessions. "I was so severely tired that I went back into the hospital to again have water drained from my system. A week later I was back doing the single one hour EECP® treatments completing the regimen over the seven week course without any problems."

Were you aware of any improvement, as you got more involved with the treatments?

"I didn't feel any changes during the first couple of weeks. As a matter of fact I did not even feel strong enough to drive to the treatment center. Family members and friends drove me to and from my appointments but here is the good news. After the first two weeks, I began feeling strong enough that I decided I could drive myself. I felt quite a bit better and not just expeditiously better. I would say, I actually felt much better. I felt incremental improvement as I continued on with the treatments. Now after the third week there was no doubt, I felt a whole lot better than I had in a very long time. I believe my completion date for the treatments was the end of October 2005. I feel better right now than I have in a few years. Last week I walked 35 minutes without having to stop. This is a far cry from where I was before I had the EECP® treatments. I had a call from Dr. Henry in December last year at which time he discussed stem cells and asked if I might want to be a candidate. I might just end up becoming a stem cell transplant patient. I might just do that." Peter has benefited from a non-invasive procedure that is available throughout the country and may bring relief to certain patients suffering from angina.

Close but no Cigar!

Joe is another of the Minneapolis Heart Institute patients who gained real benefit from EECP® treatments. Joe, did you have a heart attack? "No, I actually never had a heart attack, but I did come close. I'd have to take you back to 1997 when I was first diagnosed with heart disease. I was working out on the treadmill at the time at my gym when I felt these real bad pains in my chest. It actually felt like heartburn more than anything else and I thought for sure it was acid reflux. It would not go away and finally I asked my wife if she would call my doctor and see if we could get something for indigestion. Their response at the doctor's office was, 'get down to emergency right now!' A lot better advice than had been given Duane Gutcher on the night Duane called another doctor with his symptoms, I was thinking. Joe continues, "They reviewed my situation and immediately ordered an angiogram. This was the very first time I learned that I had multiple severe blockages. Very important to my condition and my future was what they also found out I had advanced diabetes." Did they not determine you to be a candidate for bypass? "No, they said the damage from diabetes was too extensive and too advanced to have bypass," replied Joe Vanassche.

Did members of your immediate family also have a history of diabetes? "My aunts had it and, yes, my sister has it now as well." So knowing what you learned in 1997 what became your course of action? "I joined a heart study group with Fairview Southfield, in Minnesota. This was an angiogenesis gene study to try and grow collateral bypass vessels for the heart. It made a lot of sense in my case to try the gene therapy and I stayed with the program a full two years." How did it turn out for you, the results? "There really weren't any results because after it was over, I found out I was one of the patients on the placebo and did not receive any of the medication." That is always the big concern with patients joining a randomized double blind study. You never know, not even the researchers or doctors know who is getting the placebo and who the actual drug. You had to have been pretty disappointed. "Not really, because a couple people who did receive the medication actually died. I guess it turned out all right or me after all." [This particular program was obviously halted but 9 other gene therapy programs are ongoing at different institutions using other medications and other growth factors.]

So, Joe, how did your path wind to Minnesota Heart Institute and to a meeting with Dr. Henry? "Well, they actually contacted me. They sent me a breakdown of all the programs they had going on to see if there was one I wanted to try. EECP® was on the list and it looked like the most non-invasive procedure. I believed it could be a procedure that might save my life and what did I have to lose but a little of my time. I was slightly on the heavy side and I made up my mind to lose some weight (15 lbs) during the course of the 7 week treatment period while I was doing the EECP®."

OK, Joe, you are now going through the 35 one-hour treatments. When do you start to see some indication of how well it is going? "I could actually notice a difference and started feeling better after about 3 weeks into the program." [The same amount of time that Peter Pierce had noticed his benefit. Ed, note.] What about the tread-mill workout, was there a notable difference after having had the treatments? "This may give you a pretty good idea. Before taking the treatments I had to take two or three nitros a day to make it through and after three weeks of treatment I didn't need to take any at all. I had a lot more stamina, a lot more energy. This is what I noticed most." Besides the treadmill, were there any other obvious signs of improvement? "Well, I became aware that I could walk up hills a lot easier and could perform general activities a lot better. I definitely felt the improvement. I also had spoken to other people in the program about their progress. They were getting better as well so it wasn't just me. I was told by the doctors, that the MRI they did on me after EECP® had shown a significant improvement. What are your doctors telling you today? "My current doctor said open heart could be a possible option but it would be considered as a last resort in my case. He cautioned as to the considerable risk but would leave the ultimate decision to me. Since I am doing as well as I am with medication and the improvement with EECP®, we agreed we should stay with the course we are on. I was told the years of my undiagnosed diabetes is what so extensively damaged my arteries."

You have just been presented two patient cases in which this procedure brought benefit when apparently nothing else would. This non-invasive solution may be appropriate for you or someone whose options are limited. This may be a treatment you would want to discuss with your physician. EECP®, a non-invasive procedure that was discovered more than 53 years ago at Harvard Medical School and finally received FDA approval in 1995.

Dr. Henry's discussion on prayer and healing is found in Chapter 17.

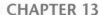

CHAPTER 13

Diabetes *and* Heart Disease

D iabetes and heart disease are both vascular diseases however, a great number of people with diabetes are not aware that the two diseases are inseparable. Diabetes complicates heart disease tremendously. The 2001 AHA article, *Diabetes Patients Are In The Dark Concerning Heart Disease* claimed that 63% of diabetic patients suffer from one or more cardiovascular complications and an alarming 80% of patients die as a result of heart disease or blood vessel disease. The report also explains that diabetes among adults increases the risk of having a heart attack or stroke two to four times. According to Sydney C. Smith, Jr., M.D., Chief Science Officer for the American Heart Association, "The AHA considers diabetes one of the major risk factors for cardio-vascular disease. Unfortunately, diabetes patients still try to treat heart disease as a separate disease."

The highly respected MUNSTER Heart Study (largest

epidemiological study done in Europe) determined that an individual with both hypertension and diabetes had an 8 times increased risk of heart attack. The two dysfunctions are commonly found in combination among diabetic patients. There are currently approximately 20.2 million Americans suffering from type II diabetes with the number up 2 million from just 3 years ago. The numbers for diabetes have actually doubled since 1980. This type of diabetes contributes to 200,000 deaths a year. Are we as a nation eating ourselves to an early appointment with the funeral home? According to the combined opinion of health organizations such as the American Diabetic Association and the American Heart Association, the answer is yes. Factors the healthcare community cites as major contributors are fast foods and the increase in restaurants serving super-sized portions of high-fat meals. Childhood obesity is rampant and schools and health educators are encouraging more daily physical exercise, less time with computer games and a diet of far less fat food. Health advocates are saying these kids aren't going to get it together by themselves. There will have to be more parental involvement, more thought invested in the preparation of family meals. How many children and adults for that matter, are getting the recommended five servings of fruits and vegetables a day and 30, 45 or 60 minutes of exercise 5 days a week? If parents have to become more active themselves in involving their children in exercise that very involvement might extend the parents' lives as well.

Statistically, there are 20.8 million children and adults in the United States currently living with diabetes and there are also 41 million unaware of their risk as "pre-diabetics." As a nation, we are looking at a total of 61.8 million people at risk.

Even though the glucose levels among many of these "pre-diabetic" individuals are not quite high enough to enter the first category of diabetes, their levels are still higher than normal. You will often hear someone say, "My doctor said I am just a little high." A "little high" should warn one of the tremendous consequences associated with being a type II diabetic and how just a little high can and will complicate the treatment and advancement of heart disease.

Diabetes Health and Medical Costs

Diabetes is an incurable disease that costs our nation over 132 billion dollars each year and accounts for more than 213,000 yearly deaths. Just the cost for the number of 54,000 amputations of lower limbs caused by ulcerated and infected legs amounts to $43,000 per amputation, a collective number of $3 billion a year. Controlling blood pressure is vitally important among diabetic patients. Among the complications that arise for diabetics is the risk of total blindness or diminished vision. When diabetes is not controlled and blood sugar levels rise, the patient is at risk for damage to the retina of the eye. There is also the risk of very painful diabetic neuropathy, which results from a destruction of the foot's sensory nerves. Diabetes Mellitus is an unforgiving disease and the sooner one is diagnosed and begins to modify the risk factors, the better the chances of controlling it. The good news coming out of the various health organizations over the past three years is the belief that diabetes, if closely monitored, can definitely be controlled. The insulin pump has been a welcomed piece of technology for many patients. It is implanted just beneath the skin and offers automatic monitoring and dispensing of just the right amount of insulin 24 hours a day.

The Good News: Diabetes is Now Considered, a Controllable Disease

What can be done to moderate the risks of diabetes? A patient who loses weight, modifies his/her diet and walks at least 30 minutes or more per day can control diabetes. Even losing 10 to 15 pounds can sometimes help bring someone out of the diabetic high risk or pre-diabetic category. The American Association of Endocrinologists provides the following list of warnings that signal the danger zone for developing diabetes, congestive heart failure and sleep apnea:

- A man's waist size exceeding 40 inches.

- A woman's waist size exceeding 35 inches.

- Blood pressure above 130/85.

- Age 45+.

• Fasting blood sugar levels over 110.

Adult Stem Cells: The Answer for Diabetes?

Marcela Valente, a reporter in Buenos Aires, Argentina reporting on a possible breakthrough in finding a cure for diabetes. According to the report, a team of doctors in Argentina used for the first time the same cell transplant approach on a diabetic as has been used in transplanting adult stem cells into heart patients. The head of the Argentinean medical team, Dr. Jorge Saslavsky, announced that the experiment involved the injection of adult stem cells into a diabetic patient, using their own stem cells. The doctors confirmed that the patient's pancreas, which had ceased to produce insulin prior to the procedure, began to function again as a result of the treatment.

The University of California at San Francisco and the University of Minnesota are doing a study involving transplantation of islet stem cells into the pancreas. In one patient whose treatment was recently completed, the need for insulin injections ceased after the transplant. The patient began producing his own insulin. There is much hope that adult stem cells may be the answer for this disease. It would certainly appear from what is already being accomplished in this area, that adult stem cells might play a major role in providing hope and remedy for this killer of people worldwide.

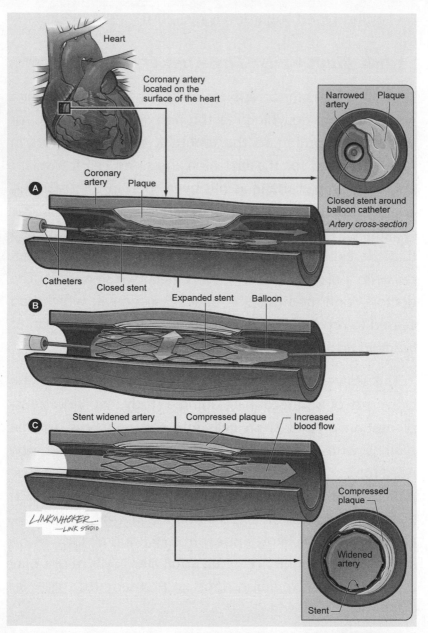

Fig. 27 Used by permission, Michael Linkinhoker, MA, CMI, of Link Studio (www.linkstudio.info) and the National Heart, Lung and Blood Institute.

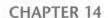

CHAPTER 14

History of
Angioplasty and
Stents

*D*r. Andreas R. Gruentzig, who died in 1985, per-formed the very first angioplasty 30 years ago in Switzerland in 1977. Dr. Gruentzig, a German radiologist, developed and performed the first successful angioplasty procedure. He took on a difficult assignment for a first attempt, opening an 80% blocked LAD (Left Anterior Descending) artery. Gruentzig, the true scientist that he was, refused to allow the press to carry the news of his first groundbreaking angioplasty until he had adequate time to perfect the process. He realized that something with such great potential for saving lives could be jeop-ardized and short lived, if too much attention were brought to the procedure before he had time to fully understand the new technology. After all, he had fash-ioned and constructed his first catheter on his own kitchen table. However, later in the same year at an American Heart Association meeting, Gruentzig presented, making public the combined results of four successful angioplastys. The first patient to have the procedure became symptom free after treatment and ten years later, when reassessed for restenosis continued to remain free. The earliest angioplasty procedures pressed the obstructive fatty deposits into the vessel wall to restore blood flow. There was, however, a 30-50% chance of failure in the original process. The fatty deposits would not remain in the position they were assigned and the artery would re-close quite readily within the first few months, necessitating a need for a second invasive procedure. The advent of angioplasty was a welcomed breakthrough in cardiovascular care, but as with any medical breakthrough there are always obstacles to overcome. Restenosis, a result of inflammation within the artery has continued through the years to be a source of reclosure of arteries following angioplasty. To mediate against this problem stent manufacturers have gone to great lengths to produce newer and more effective stents. Here are a few of the improvements that have been developed through the years, what is considered the current state of the art and what might be the next generation of stents.

The First Bare Metal Stents

In an effort to keep the fatty deposits from repositioning themselves following the procedure, the first stainless steel stent (sleeve) was developed to hold the artery open once it had been expanded. Bare metal stents were introduced in 1994 and cardiologists began using them read-ily. These stents, implemented by interventional cardiolo-gists, would render many open heart surgeries unnecce-sary and considerably reduce a good deal of the revenue stream from these surgeries to surgeons and hospitals. While the bare metal stent was an improvement, resteno-sis and reclosure of arteries continued. So what causes 30-50% of angioplastys to fail within six months? The very process of widening the artery traumatizes the artery wall and the body reacts by setting up an inflammatory response. The body, recognizing the stent as an unwel-comed foreign body, overcompensates in repair to the injured site. Once scar tissue begins to build there is a 30-50% and in some cases an 80% chance of complication with restenosis.

Medicated Stents

To help counter the inflammatory response Johnson and Johnson developed and marketed the first medicated stent. A medication on the metal stent would serve to inhibit the inflammatory response and therefore minimize the ongoing problem. Patients with diabetes are particu-larly prone to complications. Even though the advanced medicated stent was heralded as an improvement to the process, many angioplastys still continued to fail. What would replace the medicated stent and offer more long term benefit in eliminating or reducing restenosis? The scientists sharpened their pencils and went back to their drawing boards.

Drug Eluting Stents

The drug eluting stent would come to prominence in 2003. Here would be the state of the art technology, the next generation of stent. Today Americans receive 850,000 stents each year and even though bypass surgery offers a greater result in blood flow, there is much less risk of complication, infection and a lesser time to heal with angioplasty. Stents as an alternative solution to bypass surgery are an important part of the solution. Three of the major players manufacturing drug eluting stents: Cordis (Johnson & Johnson) makes the *Cypher* stent and Boston Scientific the *Taxus* stent. Medtronics has its own version called the *Endeavor* stent.

Dissolveable Stents

The recent meetings of the American College of Cardiology provide the latest news of what may possibly be a more advanced stent that is actually designed to dissolve within the artery in an allotted time after it has completed its task of keeping the artery from reclosure. This stent, still in trial, is made in part from magnesium and is biodegradable. It is believed that the dissolvable stent will provide certain advantages. One expected advantage is that the individual will still be able to have an MRI once the stent dissolves. MRI (magnetic resonance imaging) utilizes powerful magnets and a patient with a metal stent is precluded from having an MRI. Secondly, once it dissolves the foreign body is eliminated from the system.

Not Enough Angioplasties
Being Done in a Timely Manner

A consensus statement offered by the American Heart Association in 2006 cited angioplasty as the optimal treatment to open blocked vessels and restore blood flow in heart attack patients, providing it is performed in a timely manner, after the onset of symptoms. According to Dr. Alice Jacobs, former President of the AHA, today a professor of medicine and Director of the Cardiac Catherization Laboratory and Interventional Cardiology at Boston University Medical Center, "Even when patients receive primary PCI (percutaneous coronary intervention) only a minority receive the treatment within the timeframe recommended by American College of Cardiology/American Heart Association guidelines." [That timeframe, according to the guidelines, would be 90 minutes from entrance to the hospital or clinic.]

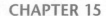

CHAPTER 15

Cedars Sinai
Catherization and
Stem Cell Program

M.D. Rajendra (Raj) Makkar is an interventional cardiologist and co-director of the Intervention Research Center and Catherization laboratory at Cedars Sinai Medical Center in Los Angeles, CA. Dr. Makkar serves as the principal investigator of several research studies including the ongoing stem cell program that utilizes bone marrow blood derived stem cells for the repair of a patient's heart following a heart attack. His leadership research roles extend to the Cypher® drug eluting stent (DES), a new generation of stent we have mentioned that promises a viable answer to the all important issue of restenosis [artery reclosure] which has occurred in about 40-50% of angioplasty procedures. As well, Dr. Makkar has helped pioneer an amazing bit of technology called the P-vad pump. A (ventricle assist device) permits the interventionalist to perform angioplasty procedures on patients whose hearts weakened from their advanced condition or age would not have otherwise been able to undergo a lengthy procedure.

A High Risk Interventional Practice

I had already been aware that the program at Cedars is designed as a high-risk interventional practice. I had also been told, "Makkar does not shy away from difficult cases." Much of his work therefore, comes through referrals by cardiologists who might feel less comfortable in tackling a particular procedure or who wish to explore options before advising a patient to go through open-heart surgery as their only solution. A well-known cardio-thoracic surgeon in Pittsburgh shared with me that if he himself needed a procedure he would want Makkar to do it.

As excited as the doctor is about the future of the ongoing cell therapy program he directs, I believed there was a wealth of additional information to be gained from this cardiologist and it would be an opportunity lost if I did not take advantage of our meeting to ask a few topical and varied questions about the process and science of angiography. These are questions I would anticipate that you, the reader, would have wanted to ask Dr. Makkar if you had been seated at our table on this particular morning. He graciously agreed to explore those questions before entering the discussion of the stem cell program. I decided to put this in a particularly reader friendly question and answer format.

Q. Dr. Makarr, you frequently use a rotar blade to prepare an artery for stenting. What is involved with this procedure?

A. The procedure is called rotational atherectomy and uses a very high-speed diamond tipped rotary burr. We use it to cut through calcified sections within an artery. Cutting through these calcified plaques is almost like cutting through cement.

Q. Now, I would imagine the most frequent follow-up question patients would want to ask you when they first hear about the procedure is, 'where do all the grindings go?' Is there risk of them independently forming a blockage?

A. We use the rotar blade to churn the calcified plaques into micro-particles; we grind the calcified areas to a very fine powdered dust that flushes out through the kidneys.

Q. A few years ago there was much promise in another form of atherectomy where the cardiologist could actually cut through the fatty plaques. This is a similar yet different procedure than the rotational atherectomy?

A. Yes it is, the atherectomy procedure you refer to is called directional atherectomy. In this procedure we actually cut loose the plaque and retrieve it as opposed to grinding it and flushing it from the body. It has failed to fulfill its promise. The problem has been restenosis, re-narrowing of the artery in the months following procedure. I do however still use it occasionally in opening leg arteries. When we do an angioplasty or in the case of the atherectomy, unfortunately neither procedure guarantees preventing re-narrowing.

Q. I have a chapter earlier in the book that deals with diabetes and heart disease. I am sure many readers would like to know what unique features you might physically see when you enter an artery of a diabetic patient.

A. When we enter the coronary arteries of a diabetic patient we are aware that these patients tend to have smaller arteries as compared to the patient who has heart disease alone. In fact, the very reason the arteries are smaller is because the plaque burden is more diffused, spreading through and affecting the larger segment of the artery wall [as opposed to being a collected blockage in one or two locations within the artery as one might find with someone who does not have diabetes.] When looking at the results of interventions with coronary angioplastys and subsequent stent procedures over the years we have learned that these procedures are not as effective in the diabetic patient, compared to what we have come to expect in the non-diabetic patient. I think that while we are equal in surgical outcomes in a number of different medical areas, the challenges we face in interventional cardiology at this point, when it comes to diabetics, is that we are somewhat limited in what we can do for them even with the newer drug eluting stents."

Q. As an interventional cardiologist, you see first-hand how heart disease and diabetes in combination complicate the process. What would be your advice for the diabetic patient or someone diagnosed as heading toward diabetes?

A. There is much that can be done for controlling diabetes in general, through diet, weight reduction, taking care of central obesity issues and certainly getting the proper amount of exercise.

Angiography

Q. You have obviously spent years understanding and teaching the principals and concepts of angiography to the professional, would you mind sharing angiography 101 with us?

A. What an angiogram actually provides is a shadow of a pipe, If you will, a two-dimensional shadow of a three dimensional structure. What I have come to learn after all the years of study and application is that the procedure is fraught with limitations. It often overestimates disease and more often underestimates disease.

Q. Many people reading what we are discussing have probably thought of the angioplasty procedure as the absolute final word in coronary artery disease detection, including its ability to identify vulnerable plaque. Are they right and how would you characterize the capabilities of the technology?

A. The angiogram does not always tell me which plaque is vulnerable. When you fill up a tube [his earlier illustration] you are seeing what is in the vessel lumen [artery center] but you are not seeing what is in the vessel wall [endothelium]. We do have the technology of interventional ultrasound (IVRUS) in which we can view the artery in a cross-sectional way and I probably use ultrasound in about 30% of my cases. [He also reminds us, ultrasound is not a non-invasive procedure.] Because the head of the catheter is large enough to accommodate a miniature camera there is a size consideration and associated risk in introducing the unit into the artery compared to the very thin wire we typically use in angiography. It is relatively more intrusive. There is a concern of dislodging plaque from the vessel wall in feeding it through the artery. You have to look at the pluses and the minuses in making a decision to use or not use interventional ultrasound. Yes, frequently angiographically, I can see features of a plaque that may have ruptured or become ulcerated but paragraphically, for every plaque you can see there may be a hundred other smaller plaques you cannot see by angiogram. Often in the past when I've looked into an artery and saw a relatively small 20% plaque, I might have told the patient everything is normal, but in fact today I tend to look at it in the opposite way. When a 20% plaque is identified, I tell the patient it is time to wake up and to become very aggressive about lifestyle changes and preventive aspects of therapy. You see, when we see a 20% plaque on an angiogram, we now know because of a phenomenon called Glagov remodeling that the plaque has already grown substantially in the vessel wall. M.D. Seymour Glagov from the University of Chicago had determined from studying arteries in autopsy specimens that the artery first enlarges on the outside of the artery to make room for a growing plaque. It is nature's way of preserving

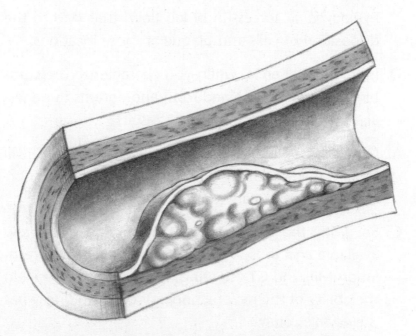

Fig. 28 An example of Galgov's principle. Illustrated by Jeeyoung.

the interior of the artery [lumen] in order to keep the blood flowing through the artery. What Dr. Glagov has shown us by his studies is that the plaque can only grow on the outside of the artery to a given point—it then has to encroach (grow) on the inside of the lumen, eventually blocking the artery."

Q. As an angiographer looking back at all the angiograms you have performed, would you say plaque burden tends to build up more frequently in a particular artery?

A. I would say not necessarily in one particular artery but more at the bifurcations [branches] in the arteries and the reason for this may be that there are local *hymodynamic* forces [in blood flow] that lead to the disposition of cells and plaque at those locations.

Q. In your experience, when you characterize the combined knowledge gained from angiograms in general, how would you qualify the results?

A. One third will require intervention, one third will require medical therapy and one third turn out normal not requiring any therapy.

Q. So, with the newest detection technologies now available and those currently in trial such as hi-resolution MRI and CT scanning, what do you foresee in the ability of the new technology compared to what is available today?

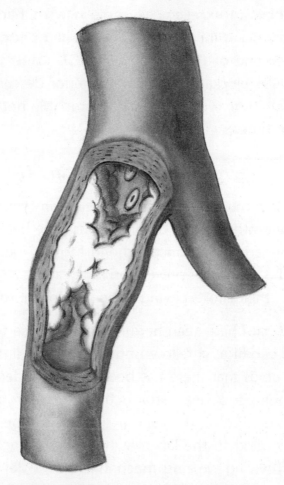

Fig. 29 Bifurcation plaque buildup. Illustrated by Jeeyoung.

A. With the current technology now available there is still difficulty in assessing the severity of lesions; however with the newer angiography with a lot of patients we will be able to more accurately rule out significant disease. This newer detection technology will prevent many needless trips to the *Cath Lab.* I think an excellent example is what happened to a physician friend of mine who had decided to go in for one of the hi-sensitivity CT scans and found a 90% blockage in his left anterior descending artery (LAD) he would otherwise probably not have found in time.

Progress in Slowing Heart Disease

Q. Over the past 7 years the American Heart Association and other health organizations have been even more engaged in a concerted effort to get the word out to the public that prevention is key, are you seeing results of their efforts paying off in your day-to-day practice?

A. What I have seen here at Cedars, since the time that I began as a fellow until today as I direct this *Cath Lab*, is that there has been a striking decrease in the number of heart attacks that come through this hospital. We used to see a greater number of patients coming to the lab that had heart attacks and were surviving wearing mechanical assist devices. We are now aware that the number has clearly and dramatically gone down. I would say the reason for the decline is due in part to very aggressive preventive therapies. However, it is not only because of statins but also because of ACE inhibitors and increased education people are getting from the articles and books they are reading like your book on prevention and treatment.

Left Main Surgery or Left Main Angioplasty?

Q. Professor Patrick Serruys, an interventional cardiologist from Erasmus University presented very positive data comparing results of left main stenting to left main bypass surgery at a meeting of the American College of Cardiology. What is the significance of this favorable comparison?

A. Until now the left main artery has traditionally been the bastion of the heart surgeon. This new device we have developed, called the P-vad heart pump, will now help many patients avoid left main artery bypass. The P-vad makes it possible for a cardiologist like myself to place a stent in the left main artery that before would have to be a case referred for surgery.

Q. How does it function?

A. It is very much like an artificial heart, I often put the patient on the P-vad pump as a support system. It is really very compact, small enough to actually fit in a person's hand. During procedure it is strapped to the patient's leg and effectively increases the heart's blood flow by a remarkable 85%. Once I can unload the heart I can then go ahead and safely do an intervention on the patient. The possibilities this device will bring to the interventional cardiologist and the additional safety factors for the elderly patient are extraordinary.

Getting to the Meat of the Meeting

Q. Dr. Makarr, when and how did the interest in stem cell therapy begin for you?

A. It actually began about five years ago after seeing some early work done by surgeons in Canada that had really fascinated me. You see, as an interventional cardiologist, I knew even though we "fix" the artery there is a reservoir of patients who will continue to experience more damage downstream. Patients who will frequently come back to the hospital repeatedly with heart failure related issues. What really piqued my interest was that one could exploit the currently available technology with the currently available biologic technology. The potential of cells in combination to what we already have available to attain additional patient benefit.

It is certainly important to be excited about the possibilities but it is also important that we as scientists can keep pace with what we can actually deliver, so nothing happens that will disappoint the public; causing them to lose interest in the field. I think that is kind of what happened with gene therapy whose potential had created a good amount of excitement. So I think we need time to better understand the basic mechanisms. We don't always understand in medicine how things work and yet the very things we don't fully understand are actually working to help patients. I believe the area of intramyocardial therapeutics, whether it is cells, growth factors or a combination of growth factors and cells, or possibly a triple combination of growth factors, cells and genes are all going to be quite relevant in treating patients with congestive heart failure in the coming years and decades. So Christian, I guess that is what really got me started. I came back from Canada very excited about what I had seen. I distinctly remember going to my collaborator's office, Michael Lill, a stem biologist, and sharing with him that I would one day like to be able to tell a patient who comes to us having had a heart attack that there is now more that we can offer them. I knew I would first have to understand much more about the technology but believed it was a time to get involved.

That visit to Canada Dr. Makkar mentioned was a little more than five years ago and in January 2006 the Cedars' cell therapy program performed its first transplant in the first patient using blood derived bone marrow stem cells.

Q. I know it is early in the program but is there anything you could share with us at this point?

A. What I can you tell you so far is that the majority of patients have benefited at four months. As a group of patients the ejection fraction has improved. I am very encouraged about this field but as a scientist I purposely refrain from over-reading the early results.

Q. Your program, as I understand, calls for injecting the patient within a short period of time after having a heart attack as compared to some approaches that accept patients whose heart attacks happened even years before. What are the parameters that guide you in your injections and therapy? What is your actual time window?

A. Our study protocol calls for cells to be injected within 3-14 days after the acute heart attack and is based in part on the protocol Andreas M. Zeiher*, M.D. used in Europe. From a practical point of view I would say that at this point we have chosen to inject from 5-14 days. I have decided to delay injecting until at least five days following the attack."

Q. There is an inflammatory response initiated by a heart attack—is that why you need to delay the injections?

A. Yes, inflammation does occur immediately and it can actually threaten the survival of the cells. On the other hand if we wait too long there is a valid argument that in the setting of an acute heart attack we may miss an opportunity, as the signals that are present at the time at the site of the infarcted heart, may potentially help differentiate these cells.

Q. After my having been in the OR (operating room) myself as an observer of actual cell transplants, I was somewhat struck by the similarity between intracoronary delivery of cells and the actual angiogram procedure. I am reminded of the cost comparison between open-heart surgery and the eventual cost of intervention in heart disease from gene and cell therapy. After doing a small amount of mathematical calculating I am just beginning to see what a colossal impact this stem therapy is going to have on the economics of health care. The vision is almost unimaginable, when one takes into account the cost of a middle aged man or woman's treatment from the point of beginning his/her management of heart disease through one or more heart attacks, open heart surgeries and hospital related visits on through final decline. When one considers the economics of bypass heart surgery at an average cost of 65K for a minimal intervention to 150K for multiple grafts to 300K for a complicated procedure and the additional costs of hospital stays, pacemakers, defibrillators and subsequent procedures, not to mention the expense of top of the line medications for 30 years, one realizes that the costs of heart disease per patient are gigantic. On the other hand, here comes a typically one-time cell transplant therapy, similar in application to an angiogram that can rebuild the heart, eventually clear the arteries and even normalize the hearts of heart failure patients.

From where I am sitting, realizing of course the medical profession is not an entirely philanthropic industry, I am wondering where will the medical profession make its money in this stem cell phenomenon? From a purely practical and economic point of view, the combined costs of a single patient from the beginning development of heart disease through the rest of their life when compared to a one-time stem cell transplant the comparison is awesome. There has not been wide exposure in the media in spite of the tremendous documented success of heart repair over the past 4 or 5 years as witnessed in the FDA studies. If one follows the money as the saying goes, is this new science going to make money for the medical profession or take away from the current revenue stream? Is there an elephant in the room? What is ahead for the medical profession?

Designer "Off the Shelf" Cells

A. I believe the future will demand more than just injecting the patient's cells. Just doing the injections is not where the profit will be for the medical profession. Even though the field of stem cell research has moved fairly quickly, I think the industry has not, at this point, fully embraced this therapy because it doesn't see much potential to get involved other than by producing a few catheters. I think, as do many of my colleagues, that the potential is there to produce "Off the Shelf Designer Cells." I believe these cells will be more specialized, more enhanced and therefore more beneficial for the patient. As I teach my fellows that train with me, the cells we are working with today are Vanilla Cells but the future will be for enhanced and improved Designer cells.

What you would have essentially would be Off The Shelf, pre-prepared product ready for injection. The theoretical argument would be that there would no longer be a need to do a bone marrow tap on the patient, as these cells would be readily available to be ordered and administered just like any drug. The time to prepare and expand patient's cells would as well, no longer be required. Here would be the the-oretical appeal or advantage if you will, of a business angle that the industry would potentially use to become more involved.

* *Dr. Zeiher is one of the pioneers in stem cell research and a former colleague of Dr. Makkar's having earleir been in the Cedars' fellow-ship program.*

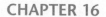

CHAPTER 16

Johns Hopkins
Stem Cell Program

J oshua Hare, M.D., Director of Heart Failure and
Cardiac Transplantation and Director of the
Cardiovascular section in The Institute for Cell
Engineering at The Johns Hopkins University School of
Medicine (JHU), asserts, "What we at Johns Hopkins and
the other scientists and researchers at other facilities are
all addressing is a completely unmet need to create the
ability to regenerate heart tissue. To do that, we are using
a variety of cell approaches for a variety of heart diseases.
We realize there is still a long way to go. A lot of refinement will need to be done."

When I spoke with the director he had just returned from
informative meetings and presentations of the latest session
of the American Heart Association. He described the collec-
tive progress that was represented there. "Stem cell technology and science have now reached a pivotal point, as
the two areas continue to press forward. While enthusiasm

is good, there is still a lot of work ahead in proving technologies beyond the lab and into the real world environment." Dr. Hare continues, "there are a lot of very exciting things going on in the basic science labs and a good amount of transitional work is guiding the therapies that are being developed—even though we are, at this time, not yet able to jump directly into the therapeutic arena"

Dr. Hare and his colleagues At JHU are working with a specific form of bone marrow stem cell technology called mesenchymal. (me-sen-chy-mal) stem cells. "These adult cells are also non-embryonic bone marrow stem cells which have shown in earlier animal studies to have the potential for repairing damaged hearts." Last year, Dr. Hare's research in animals showed that stem cells harvested from a pig's bone marrow and injected into another pig's damaged heart restored heart function and repaired damaged heart muscle by 50 to 75 percent. In March 2005 Dr. Hare and other researchers began a Phase I clinical trial to test the safety of injecting adult stem cells at varying doses in patients who had recently suffered a heart attack. In total, 48 patients are participating in this study, which involves several sites across the country, including JHU. As doctor Hare was quoted earlier in this book as saying, "bone marrow transplants for the heart may be new but bone marrow treatment therapy has been used in fighting diseases like leukemia and lymphoma for years."

What is Different About Mesenchymal Cells?

Dr. Hare, "These mesenchymal cells are very versatile, besides being used for the heart they also have the capacity to be used in the treatment of many other diseases as well." What other diseases would you anticipate might one day benefit from the ongoing JHU studies? "Certainly in myocardial infarction, in different kinds of bone diseases and cartilage disease. These cells also affect the immune system so they have the potential to work in graft verses host disease." Do you foresee a potential for eventually treating neuromuscular disease? "Possibly, these cells may have greater capacity than we had actually anticipated. There is also the possibility these cells may send a chemical signal to other cells that are already present in the body. If this does happen, it might actually increase the healing capacity of these cells. They also have an ability to home (seek) to areas of injury in need of repair."

The Big Picture

"What is so exciting about the work in progress right now" says Director Hare, "is that a number of cellular regenerative approaches are being studied at various medical centers that have actually made it into the testing stage. The progress made so far has moved us forward to the place where we are now in the actual clinic performing the studies, proving these technologies for the public's benefit. To do that, we are using a variety of cell approaches for a variety of heart diseases. We realize there is still a long way to go. A lot of refinement will need to be done." Richard Lange, Chief of Clinical Cardiology at Hopkins who leads research efforts in ischemic heart disease and adult congenital heart disease has said, "This is an incredibly exciting time to be working in cardiac care because we are at the forefront of some key medical breakthroughs, including research on a first-ever cure for heart attack in humans, a discovery that would change cardiac care as we know it today."

When is a Stem Cell a Stem Cell?

Dr. Hare explains, "A true stem cell has the capacity to self renew. A true stem cell can differentiate into different lineages" (varieties). How would you describe the difference between muscle skeletal cells and bone marrow cells? "In comparison, skeletal cells can only serve the one purpose they were designed to do and that purpose is to turn into skeletal muscle. It may be just a matter of semantics, but a skeletal cell is not in the true sense a stem cell. There is a slight difference between being a skeletal [precursor cell] and a stem cell."

Your Magnificent Heart

The heart is an incredible piece of machinery. To appreciate what it does it might be interesting to understand how it functions. The heart has four chambers with the command center positioned in the right atrium. The purpose of the command center is actually to control the critical electrical impulses that dictate the timing of contractions to all chambers of the heart. A "misfire" may offset the natural rhythm of the chambers, producing a catastrophic affect. Not unlike your automobile that misfires, lunges and jerks until it finally stalls. The atrium sends electrical signals to the two lower chambers, the left and right ventricles that then accept and pump blood to the rest of the body. Anything that interferes with this rhythmic ballet can cause the heart, as your automobile engine, to stutter and stall.

Cardiac Arrest / Sudden Death

Cardiac arrest is most often the result of suspected or even unsuspected heart disease. In 90% of cases, two or more major coronary arteries have been compromised by atherosclerosis. Sudden death, as the term suggests, can strike without warning and in many cases is the final result of heart failure. The AHA advocates an immediate call to 911 and the beginning of CPR; time is of the essence, as the patient's chance of survival without intervention will decrease 7-10% with each passing minute. If emergency services arrive within 5-7 minutes to begin defibrillation, there is an approximate 49% success rate in reviving the victim. Sudden death is sometimes referred to as sudden cardiac arrest or unexpected cardiac arrest.

Here are the study statistics presented at the American Heart Association's 41st Annual Conference on Cardiovascular Disease, Epidemiology and Prevention. Cardiac arrest remains the cause of 259,000 deaths a year in this country alone. One half of those who die of heart disease succumb within one hour of the noticeable symptoms. Twenty-five to thirty-three percent of those who suffer sudden cardiac death die instantly, and unless the event has occurred in the presence of others, the victim is usually found after the fact quite by accident. The remaining patients, who experience symptoms and are able to get to a hospital to take advantage of emergency care, are the lucky ones. The statistics report that about one half of CHD deaths each year are attributed to sudden death cases, accounting for more than 680 people per day. The AMA and the AHA advise learning the symptoms and not hesitating to act if you or someone you know are displaying symptoms. Have someone take you to the hospital ASAP or call paramedics. It would not be wise to go to sleep waiting to see if the symptoms are still there in the morning. It is possible that something as simple as indigestion may ultimately turn out to be the cause; however, many people have delayed seeking medical attention, misdiagnosing their own symptoms, with great detriment to themselves.

Avoiding the Heart Lung Machine

While open-heart surgery has beyond a doubt saved millions of lives, the very idea and mandate of preventive medicine is to do the things necessary to avoid ever becoming a heart disease patient who would require so dramatic an invasive procedure. There remains the fact that many patients who undergo open heart (particularly when using the heart lung machine) have shown a 42% decline in certain cognitive functions over the years following the operation. Operations done on a beating heart produce a much less negative result and researchers are working on new ways to eliminate some of the negative aspects of open-heart surgery. One of the concerns is the calcification present at the place where the heart lung machine connects at the aorta. Particles of the calcified plaque break loose and migrate through the arteries over time to lodge finally in the vessels of the brain. Cardiologists have been puzzled over how many patients who did well during the first six months following surgery became symptomatic and displayed personality changes and cognitive dysfunction over the next 4, 5 or 6 years. Applying a small filter at the aorta is one technique being studied. The beating heart operation has the advantage for the patient in keeping adequate blood flow and oxygen over a sometimes-long period under anesthesia. As everyone knows, open-heart surgery is a highly invasive procedure, which can be even more traumatic when the patient, 15 or 20 years later, must face a second or third surgery in poorer health than the first time. Wouldn't it be an advance to offer senior patients who find themselves in this situation an alternative solution—a viable non-invasive alternative?

CHAPTER 17

Prayer and the *Minneapolis Heart Institute* Study

*I*n recalling their heart attack experiences, you may have noticed how several of the patient's stories you have just read expressed how important their belief system and spiritual connection was in getting them through their crises. The subject of spirituality and prayer did in fact find itself very much at home in the conversation as expressed by the patients. Was this a coincidence; was the interest a result of pre-conditioning or is there more to the connection? When someone comes very close to the final curtain, does the subject more fervently present itself? It would seem so. We've probably never heard it so well expressed than in the saying, "There are no atheists on deathbeds or in foxholes." Laurance Johnston, Ph.D, made this comment, "Almost everyone prays when faced with a traumatic injury like spinal cord injury (SCI) or a debilitating disease such as multiple sclerosis (MS)." No doubt we would include heart attacks as well. When the emotional need is great, as it is during any national crisis or when one's own health is failing, people who might have never looked upward before are suddenly down on their knees.

THE GOD GENE was the cover title of a *Time Magazine*, October 24, 2004. Interestingly, the cover also carried the following text, "Does our DNA compel us to seek a higher power?" The cover information answered it's own question, 'Believe it or not, some scientists say yes.' When Dr. Harold Koenig, a Professor of Psychiatry and Co-director for the Center for Spirituality, Theology and Health at Duke University, was asked by a reviewer to comment on the article, he replied, "There is some research suggesting that humans actually are biologically wired to be religious or spiritual."

When I asked Dr. Tim Henry if he would summarize what has been learned thus far from the Minneapolis Prayer Study he currently oversees at the Heart Institute, he replied, "We have found that patients who have a positive spiritual outlook tend to do better than patients who do not." Dr. Deepak Chopra, who has been outspoken on the connection between science and spirituality. "It is just as I have contended all along, there are healing forces in nature that science is only now just beginning to understand." Dr. Koenig comments, "Religion has a power to heal, and we have an obligation to value that alongside of medicine." Perhaps no one ever expressed it better than the great man of science himself in splitting the baby both ways, "Science without religion is lame.

Religion without science is blind."—Albert Einstein.

A quick review of the literature reveals that there has been an ongoing concerted interest in these phenomena of prayer and healing for thousands of years and today the interest is only growing. As example, ten years ago only three of the nation's medical schools carried courses in their curriculum for prayer and spirituality. Today, seventy-nine of America's 125 medical schools offer classes in healing and prayer. There have been more than 1,200 studies done on the subject at such prestigious academic and governmental institutions as Harvard, Columbia, the CDC, World Health Organization, Institutes of Health, UCLA and the Mayo Clinic.

Can prayer actually help one's health? According to Dr. Koenig, "Substantial scientific evidence indicates, yes. Patients who have been in the studies who pray and have a certain kind of belief system, have lower blood pressure and a lowered incidence of stroke and heart disease." Laurance Johnston, Ph.D., whose work with complimentary and alternative medicine is legendary, voiced his views on this subject of prayer in his piece *Prayer is Making a Medical Comeback*. He writes, "Given that 94% of Americans believe in God or a higher power (1994 Gallup Poll), it is not surprising that 75% of patients think that their physician should address spiritual issues as part of their medical care. Furthermore, 40% want their physicians to actively discuss religious issues with them and nearly 50% want their physicians to pray not just for them, but also with them. In a growing trend, 43% of American physicians privately pray for their patients. An article in the *Journal of the American Medical Association* (JAMA, May 1995) entitled, *Should Physicians Prescribe Prayer for Health?* discussed these trends. The mere presence of this article in this highly respected bastion of the medical profession suggests that the barrier between spirituality and health care is crumbling" said the reviewer.

A Harris Poll put another touch on the religion and healing issue recently when they submitted their survey findings enlisted from 2,306 adults. Their finding was that only 9% of those polled did not believe in God. Forty three percent of the physicians polled by Gallup said they actually pray privately for their patients. And, no, I don't think they are praying for patients to pay their bills.

When Science and Religion Coexist

Dr. Farr Curlin from the Center for Medical Ethics, Department of Medicine at the University of Chicago, "We did not think physicians were nearly this religious." Of 1,044 doctors interviewed from across the country, 59% said they believe in some kind of afterlife and 55% percent said their religious beliefs influence how they practice medicine. But the finding that surprised Dr. Curlin the most among these men of science, was that 76% said they believed in God. "We were surprised to find that physicians were as religious as they apparently are. Dr. J. Edward Hill, President of the American Medical Association says "religion and medicine are completely compatible, as long as doctors do not force their own beliefs on patients." The Minneapolis Heart Institute Study and its Director, Dr. Henry's comments are worth repeating, "We have found that patients who have a positive spiritual outlook, tend to do better than patients who do not." The *Power of Prayer in Medicine* was an article by Mitchell W. Krucoff, MD, Director of the Ischemia Monitoring Laboratory at Duke University Medical Center in Durham, NC and published in the American Heart Journal November 2001. This study was designed to evaluate the progress of heart patients who had people praying for them, as compared to those who did not have the benefit of prayer. Each of the patients enrolled in the study had a history of serious heart problems, and were scheduled to undergo coronary angioplasty. Dr. Krucoff says, "This was a very rigorously controlled study; we looked at the information just as we would look at any therapeutic, as with a new cardiovascular drug or a new stent, seeing the results in terms of patient outcomes." Those patients for whom others had been praying for showed significantly fewer complications than the other patients who had not received prayers. Prayer and spirituality are very personal matters but the information presented here in this chapter on spirituality and prayer would indicate that the great majority of Americans do recognize God as a source of strength in times of health crisis and that heart patients in particular benefit from prayer.

CHAPTER 18

Growing *Portfolio* *of Other* *Adult Cell* *Successes*

Stem Cells for Diabetes

At both the University of Minnesota and the University of California at San Francisco, islet stem cells are being successfully injected into the pancreas of a type I diabetes patient. The first patient to have the one-time islet transplant has remained insulin free for a year. The program is now recruiting other candidates.

Stem Cells for the Eyes

M.D. Edward Holland from the Cincinnati Eye Institute operated on a young man named Todd Heritage and helped him regain his sight using stem cells from a living relative. He has performed several successful cell transplants.

Stem Cells for Macular Degeneration

The number one cause of blindness among citizens over age 55 is macular degeneration affecting 1.75 million Americans. There is reason to believe stem cells can offer some hope for these patients according to the senior author of a study done at Florida University. Edward Scott, Ph.D., a professor of molecular genetics at UF Shands Cancer Center and director of the Program In Stem Cell Biology and Regenerative Medicine. "What this tells us, is for problems such as age related macular degeneration, we should be able to harvest cells to help repair the damage." The researchers at UF believe it may be possible to also grow new cells in the retina to replace cells lost to injury or disease.

Stem Cells for Lungs

Researchers at the University of Minnesota are using progenitor cells harvested from cord blood to differentiate them into alveolar [respiratory] cells "Turning a cord blood stem cell into an alveolar cell represents a significant milestone in stem cell research. Though further research is needed, it's plausible, the Multi-Lineage Progenitor Cell (MLPC) from cord blood could be used to help develop a human lung model for research purposes and/or eventual therapeutic application to treat a number of respiratory conditions – such as emphysema and pulmonary fibrosis as well as pulmonary injury due to therapy–related causes." David McKenna, M.D., assistant professor of Lab Medicine and Pathology.

Stem Cells for Neurodegenerative Disease

Neurodegenerative diseases include Multiple Sclerosis and Parkinson's disease. The study authors from the Felenstein Medical Research Center and Department of Neurology at Rabin Medical Center, the Sackler School of Medicine, Tel Aviv University in Israel, have concluded, "These mesenchymal (bone marrow) stem cells (MSC's) are predisposed to differentiate into neuronal cells given the proper conditions. When transplanted into the central nervous system, they will develop into a variety of functional neural cell types, making them a potent resource for cell-based therapy."

Stem Cells for Cancer

Vanderbilt University has performed their first transplant using umbilical cord stem cells for treating a patient with cancer. The City of Hope is curing some forms of cancer with adult bone marrow stem cells. There are no less than 30 ongoing cancer trials treating a wide variety of cancers, including malignant brain tumors and breast cancer using adult stem cells. There are currently 562 government adult stem cell trials in progress.

Stem Cells for Kidney Disease

Stem cells derived from bone marrow appear to reverse genetic kidney disease, researchers at Beth Israel Deaconess Medical Center said they successfully used stem cells to regenerate damaged renal cells in an animal model of a genetic kidney disorder known as Alport syndrome.

Stem Cells for Spinal Injury Repair

Spinal injury repair and neurodegenerative diseases have until now been considered an area that would only benefit from embryonic stem cells however, researchers at the UC Irvine Reeve-Irvine Research Center have used adult human neural stem cells to successfully regenerate damaged spinal cord tissue and improve mobility in mice. The findings point to the promise of using this type of cells for possible therapies to help humans who have spinal cord injuries. *Source: Proceedings of the National Academy of Sciences.*

World famous animal trainer-entertainer Roy Horn, of Siegfried and Roy, has now been able to walk short steps three years after the devastating spinal injury he suffered when his favorite tiger attacked him during a nightly Las Vegas show. Roy, in a last attempt to find a cure, flew to Germany for stem cell treatments. As a result of the treatments, the entertainer is beginning to walk again. Dr. Albert Scheller told the German Press Agency prior to Roy Horn's transplantation, "Horn is undergoing stem cell therapy using cells from his own body." Scheller explained, the "stem cells are removed from cartilage in the patient's knee." According to John Katsilometes, a Las Vegas Sun writer, "Roy can walk, unaided, short distances."

Stem Cells for Sickle Cell

Doctors in France announced they believe they can cure children with severe sickle cell disease through stem cell transplants without risking serious complications or death. The researchers, who have performed 69 transplants since 1988, reported an 85% disease-free survival.

A New Gene Discovery

A gene called "nanog" appears to be the most important among several "reprogramming genes" that could transform adult stem cells into an embryonic-like state. According to research published in the June 14, 2006 online edition of the journal *Nature*, Jose Silva and colleagues from the University of Edinburgh's Institute for Stem Cell Research have found the pathway by which embryonic stem cells obtain "pluripotency." Pluripotency allows the cells to develop into more than 200 cell types found in the body.

CHAPTER 19

Coenzyme Q10
necessary with all
Statin Drug Intake

C oenzyme Q10 (obiquinone) is a vitamin-like nutrient critically important to all heart disease patients. Karl Folkers, Professor Emeritus, was in the 1980's Vice-President for Exploratory Research for the pharmaceutical giant Merck. At that time the company was in development of lovestatin (Mevacor®), the first cholesterol-lowering drug that would come to market in 1987. Dr. Folkers had found in earlier studies that Coenzyme Q10 was vital to heart muscle strength and that a deficiency in the body's production of the enzyme would weaken the heart muscle. Also, what is heart failure but a condition in which the heart loses strength and ability to pump? Earlier studies had determined, Coenzyme Q10 to be deficient among heart failure patients. He informed his company that while indeed their statin drug effectively lowered cholesterol, it did it at a cost of inhibiting the body's natural production of Coenzyme Q10. He warned that Co

Q10 would have to be supplemented with their statin drug in order to offset the created deficiency. He must have made his point well because Merck filed not one, but two government patents that granted the company the exclusive right to produce and market a combination of Co Q10 along with their new statin drug. Merck actually drew their patents to cover Q10 in excessive amounts up to 1,000 mgs. This patent precluded any other statin manufacturer from adding the enzyme to their statin drug and competing with their sales.

In an interesting bit of irony, Merck never informed the public of the importance of taking the enzyme as protection and secondly they never exercised their own patent provision to combine it with their drug. These are the two patent numbers filed in the United States Patent and Trademark Office: 4929437 & 4933165: both are easily accessible through the government website.

In Merck's Own Words

The following is a copy of the actual text offered by Merck in making their case to obtain the exclusive right to manufacture their statin drug in combination with Coenzyme Q10. The patent application patent number is 4,933,165: As the text indicates, the manufacturer knew full well of the need to include Coenzyme Q10 with their drug and furthermore, that without the addition of the enzyme myopathy could be the consequence. Are you or someone you know not aware of the importance of this enzyme with any statin intake?

> *A pharmaceutical composition comprising a pharmaceutical carrier and an effective antihypercholesterolemic amount of an HMG-CoA reductase inhibitor [statin] and an amount of Coenzyme Q10 effective to counteract HMG-CoA reductase inhibitor-associated skeletal muscle myopathy. A method of counteracting HMG-CoA reductase inhibitor-associated skeletal muscle myopathy is a subject in need of such treatment which comprises the adjunct administration of a therapeutically effective amount of an HMG-CoA reductase inhibitor and an effective amount of Coenzyme Q10 to counteract said myopathy.*

Folkers, disappointed in his company's lack of interest in devoting more attention to this vital nutrient, relinquished his position at Merck and became President and Chief Executive Officer of Stanford Research Institute in Palo Alto, California and would eventually move to Austin, Texas to become Director of Biochemical Engineering at Texas State University. It is important to understand the quality of his credentials because what he discovered 45 years ago is finally now being acknowledged as important to your health or that of anyone taking one of the statin drugs including Lipitor®, Crestor®, Lescol®, Zocor®, Pravachol®, and Mevacor®.

Heart Failure Improvement with Coenzyme

Because of the importance in addressing this vital heart failure issue, the following information is offered in a study conducted by Dr. Folkers which determined: When Coenzyme Q10 was added to the diets of cardiomyopathy (enlarged heart) patients the same patients showed improvement. The heart muscle itself actually showed signs of improved strength. With regard to symptomatic fatigue, palpitations and chest pain, the ejection fraction showed a consistent and sustained improvement among the heart failure patients taking the supplement compared to those on placebo. Incredibly, some patients, early in their disease, actually experienced a return to their normal heart size.

Ejection Fraction Improvement in 84% of the Study Participants

The findings of Chief of Cardiology of the Manchester Hospital Coenzyme Study Steven T. Sinatra, M.D., F.A.C.C., F.A.C.N., C.N.S., Nov. 1997, demonstrate an improvement in the patients' quality of life as well as their rate of survival. Participants showed both systolic and diastolic function improvement attributable to Q10 therapy. Most important was the finding that Coenzyme Q10 had actually produced POSITIVE RESULTS AMONG VERY ADVANCED HEART PATIENTS WHEN ALL PREVIOUS TRADITIONAL MEDICAL THERAPY HAD FAILED. The study recommended that Q10 be included with traditional medicine in adjunctive therapy. This is nothing short of revolutionary!

Does Coenzyme Q10 Improve Patient Survival Rates?

When Dr. Langsjoen and Dr. Whitaker evaluated heart failure patients over three years, 75% of those on Q10 therapy, along with their normal prescriptions, survived. Of those study subjects who had not added the supplement to their medications, only 25% remained alive at the end of the study three years later. Clearly, an improvement was noted when Q10 was taken. When the study applicants who had been on conventional monolithic therapy were compared to those who were administered both conventional therapy and the coenzyme supplement, the group whose regimen included Coenzyme Q10 showed an improved survival rate! Based on this study and the evidence provided by the Sinatra and Folker's studies, what would be the reason not to prescribe heart patients the protection afforded by Coenzyme Q10?

Natural Adjuvants for Treatment of Congestive Heart Failure

A clinical research report published in *Medical Hypotheses* April 1996, supported earlier findings in regard to certain vitamins helpful for heart disease and heart failure patients. Included in this category along with Coenzyme Q10 (which we have already discussed at length) were taurine, magnesium, potassium, chromium,

L-carnitine and fish oil. The conclusion found that since these supplements come from nutritional sources, they would (as certain previous studies agreed) carry little or no toxic effect. The report suggested that there was little reason why this benefit from the combination of the various supplements just listed should not be studied as a comprehensive nutritional beneficial therapy for congestive heart failure. CHF is a very serious condition and regardless of the promising claims of researchers and physicians, your own doctor should evaluate the information with you in considering the evidence for combination therapy. Nevertheless, the information in favor of Coenzyme Q10 is nothing short of miraculous.

Coenzyme Q10 Link to Congestive Heart Failure

There has been a dramatic increase in congestive heart failure cases over the past 16 years since the introduction of cholesterol lowering drugs. Many studies have implicated the wide use of statin drugs during this period as contributing to the unprecedented increase in heart failure cases. The results of a study appearing in the *American Journal of Cardiology* November 2004 indicate and support a link between heart failure and statin therapy. Peter Langsjoen M.D., F.A.C.C., a 17 year practicing cardiologist from Tyler Texas and recognized expert in statin-induced Co Q10 depletion announced the following findings: Fourteen non-heart disease patients whose primary physicians were about to start them on Lipitor therapy were enrolled. All participants were under age 50 and qualified under the National Cholesterol Education guidelines for beginning statin therapy. Each would be administered 20 mgs each day of Lipitor and remain on the regimen for 3-6 months. A standard echocardiogram was given at the beginning and end of the study. Dr. Langsjoen reported that 71% of the study patients (10 of 14) developed deficiency in heart performance. Ten of the 14 had a decrease in left ventricle function. Nine of the 10 (who had been found deficient) were then given increased amounts of Co Q10 for the following 3 months while they continued to take Lipitor®. The amount of Co Q10 had been increased from 20 mgs to 300 mgs a day.

Eight of the 9 patients (almost 90%) had a reversal of at least one of the markers of diastolic insufficiency and remarkably 44% showed improvement and reversal in all three diastolic markers of abnormality. Conclusions: As the report found, 7 of the 9 patients taking Coenzyme Q10 along with the statin drug had excellent increases in their levels of Co Q10. The study results indicate that left ventricle (pumping chamber) can have improved function when adequate Co Q10 supplementation is taken along with a statin drug. Besides the Canadian warnings there are petitions currently before the FDA in this country.

Canada Convinced, Orders Warnings

The following changes in statin drug labeling have

now been added to every statin prescription sold in Canada. The mandatory warnings were announced in the *New England Journal of Medicine* (Canadian edition) in November 2005. The following text is what now actually appears in all prescription bottles of statin drugs sold in Canada. The following language is as it is presented in the Lipitor® customer insert.

Statin Depleting Effect on Obiquinone (Coenzyme Q_{10})

Significant decreases in circulating obiquinone levels in patients treated with atorvastatin and other statins have been observed. A clinical significance of a potential long-term statin induced deficiency of obiquinone [Co Q_{10}] has not been established. It has been reported that a decrease in myocardial obiquinone levels could lead to impaired cardiac function in patients with borderline congestive heart failure. Author's note: Could it be entirely possible that term use of a statin may actually be the reason a patient becomes a borderline congestive heart failure patient in the first place as the following study implies?

How Much Coenzyme
To Counteract Statin Depletion?

According to Dr. Karl Folkers, from his initial findings, 100 mgs of Coenzyme Q10 daily was enough to reverse the detrimental side effects associated with statin therapy. The Whitaker petition before the FDA suggests a larger dosage of 100-200 mgs of coenzyme Q10 daily. How many doctors are checking their patients' levels of coenzyme while prescribing any of the HMG-CoA reductase inhibitor drugs? Are you yourself on a cholesterol lowering statin drug? Coenzyme Q10 is administered as standard protective therapy in Japan and in Europe and now suggested in Canada. You have read that a petition is now before the FDA here in the states, would you think it wise to include Coenzyme Q10 with statin intake in your own regimen?

Two Petitions Calling for Statin Warnings
in the US

Dr. Julian Whitaker, whose Whitaker Wellness Center was established in La Jolla CA in 1979 and whose newsletter reaches more than 500,000 readers, has filed two petitions with the FDA Commissioner's Office. The text of the Whitaker petition calling for mandatory warnings in the United States in an effort to protect the millions of statin drug users here, reads as follows:

Warning: HMG CoA reductase inhibitors block the endogenous biosynthesis of an essential cofactor, Coenzyme Q_{10}, required for energy production. A deficiency of Coenzyme Q_{10} is associated with impairment of myocardial function, with liver dysfunction and with myopathies (including cardiomyopathy and congestive heart failure). All patients taking HMG CoA reductase inhibitors should therefore be advised to take 100 to 200 mg per day of supplemental Coenzyme Q_{10}.

CHAPTER 20

A Remedy for Stable and Unstable Angina?

The Greeks and the Italians described the discomfort in the chest with two words. Ankhon which is a Greek word describing (strangulation) and the Latin word (pectus) for chest. Together the words describe a heart that is literally crying out in pain. William Heberden introduced the first description of angina pectoris to the medical community as he addressed the Royal College of Physicians in 1768. So much for the claim that heart disease is a product of the 20th century. Angina Pectoris (angaa-na) is an ischemic condition caused by progressive atherosclerosis, which ultimately affects blood flow to the heart. In this symptomatic stage, narrowed arteries are literally choking off the heart muscle of oxygen carrying blood. When asked to describe their symptoms, many patients will chose the word discomfort rather than describing it as actual pain, referring to the symptom as a pressure, squeezing, a heaviness or choking, or possibly a burning sensation. Episodes of angina distress may only last for a brief 1 to 5 minutes. During these times of episode the patient needs to immediately seek rest and cessation from their activity. In order to gain some relief a patient might turn to their prescriptions of nitroglycerin or other anti-angina medications. A patient who would continue being active at the time of experiencing symptoms could very likely be courting an actual heart attack. Immediate rest from physical exertion or emotional stress is a must.

The Annual Cost to the Health Care System

Different health organizations arrive at different figures and most organizations do not automatically do yearly assessments. However in 2000, six years ago 7 million patients were believed affected with angina. The estimated annual cost for the care these patients received amounted to $15 billion. Another $5 billion was estimated for outpatient medical costs. When the supportive services for this disease were added to the equation, the dollar loss of productivity to the workforce reached an estimated $40 billion! Here is a total hard number combined cost of $60 billion a year! The need to find an acceptable alternative is not only crucial for the obvious health reasons but for the economic impact as well. There is some temporary help provided by EECP® which we have earlier discussed and an emerging technology called TMR (transmyocardial revascularization), an extreme surgical measure that involves surgery and the use of a laser to open channels in the heart to increase blood flow. The greatest hope for angina patients however, lies in the potential and promise of adult stem cells. It is a cutting edge topical discussion of which few people are aware.

Will the Answer for Angina Come from Stem Cells?

Dr. Douglas Losordo, Chief of Research at St. Elizabeth's Hospital in Boston is leading the first FDA angina stem cell trial. His mission is to try and prove the benefit of adult CD4 autologous stem cells derived from the patient's own blood in bringing hope and remedy to the hundreds of thousands of patients who will have no hope. To help us better understand the ongoing trial expectations the doctor described the patient population that he and his team are working with in trying to find a solution to a disease that according to the American Heart Association, gains approximately 250,000 recruits every year.

Dr. Losordo explained, "When you look at this particular patient population with intractable angina (does not respond to available treatment) it is important to acknowledge that these are basically no option patients. Let me give you an example of how a patient in this category is identified. On more than one occasion I have assigned a medical assistant or a resident student to evaluate a new patient's health profile and history. It is not at all uncommon for the student to report that the patient, (who was here because of angina) did not actually report having chest pain. When I do a follow-up with the very same patient, I might learn the reason they are not having chest pain is simply because they have become almost totally inactive in order to avoid it. As one lady told me, "I just sit in a chair most all the time so I won't have to deal with the pain." "These patients," said Dr. Losordo, "have simply learned to fly beneath the radar screen. I have heard many of them say that after a long time living with their ailment they actually get tired of hearing themselves complain; they have just adjusted to their condition. They modify their life style and do very little to aggravate symptoms. I share this example to stress the point that while these patients are free of symptoms they are also paying a price by having to restrict their activity. Even a trip to the mailbox or to the back yard can be a challenge."

What is the Future for Angina Patients?

Doctor Losordo explained, "We have estimated that there is a special category of around 250,000 of these patients in the US, who become classified as having intractable angina. When we searched a national database we found that about a quarter million patients had been rejected for a third coronary bypass operation. This doesn't mean that those patients necessarily all fall into the intractable angina category. It would make sense however, that because they did actually present themselves for a third bypass surgery their condition had to have been serious. The very fact that they were rejected for bypass would most likely also mean that they would have already tried or been excluded from qualifying for balloon angioplasty. These patients would have exhausted all medical options available, prior to being referred for the extreme solution."

Reporting Early Study Results

Researchers from Caritas St. Elizabeth's Medical Center in Boston, Scripps Clinic of La Jolla, California and the Minneapolis Heart Institute announced very promising results from the first phase of the first U.S. clinical trial investigating adult CD4 stem cells for angina patients. Dr. Losordo, in addressing the American Heart Association meeting in Dallas Texas:

"Over the past two years 24 patients suffering from disabling angina attacks (the most severe form of chest pain) participated in the randomized, double-blind FDA-approved study. After six months of follow-up, more than 80% or 15 of the 18 patients who received the autologous adult stem cells, reported feeling better with reductions in chest pain and improved exercise capacity."

The report continued, "Generally in a Phase I pilot study we are limited to assessing the safety of the protocol since the number of patients included is generally too small to make conclusions regarding a treatment effect."

Dr. Losordo added, "We were very pleasantly surprised to learn that the autologous adult stem cells were not only well tolerated, but also appeared to show evidence of benefit. While this is very early in the clinical trial process, we are cautiously optimistic as we move into a 150-patient, national multi-site Phase II trial early in 2006."

Since no therapy has ever addressed this particular patient population the question rose, how do we measure the true effect of a therapy like this? We are being very careful and thoughtful about determining the right criteria. Should it be blood flow, is it exercise time, is there some other measurement to apply like MRI, PET scanning, or some other technique we should be using and relying on to make the final assessment? All of these things we will be looking at in Phase II.

Stable Angina or Unstable Angina

STABLE ANGINA: A patient's angina can be aggravated by anything that puts an additional workload on the heart. Certainly an emotional upset, an argument or receiving bad news will cause an increase in heart rate. The simple act of dining or being in cold weather can bring about a reaction and trigger a symptomatic response. The kind of angina that fits the above description is passive. These patients will normally find relief if they rest or rely on their medications. Therefore, the patient whose condition (in the short term) becomes stabilized may be classified as having stable angina.

UNSTABLE ANGINA: Patients whose symptoms last more than 15 minutes and did not result from the activities as those for stable angina may be diagnosed as having the more serious unstable angina. This latter condition is more advanced and is more likely to bring the patient to the ER most frequently for hospitalization, according to the American Heart Association.

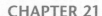

CHAPTER 21

ACE Inhibitors, Life Saving Miracle Drugs

*A*n ACE inhibitor is a vasodilator class of drug that reduces the workload of the heart by widening the artery channel, thereby increasing the degree of blood flow. Angiotensin is a substance produced by the body that instead of opening the channel actually narrows it. Therefore, for the heart patient, it is advisable to reduce angiotensin. The life saving attributes of this drug does not stop there.

Heart Failure and ACE Inhibitors

According to an Aug. 2004 article appearing in the journal *Circulation of The American Heart Association*, "Almost a third of heart failure patients face an increased risk of death because they do not receive an angiotensin-converting enzyme (ACE) inhibitor." Dr. John Kennedy, a cardiologist at Glasgow Nuffield Hospital commenting on the study summed it up this way, "Ace inhibitors are currently under-prescribed and often used in inadequate doses." Professor James Mathew and colleagues at the University of Iowa College of Medicine carried out the study on ACE inhibitors and heart failure. Dr. Mathew calls for patients to be tested for heart muscle thickening using an echocardiogram (ECG) test. "We think, we can now reduce the risk of cardiovascular events and death by regression of left ventricular hypertrophy using ECG markers." Dr. Mathew, based on his findings, concluded, "Until now, no agent [referring to the ACE drug Remipril (Altace®)] has been shown to lower risk by causing a regression of left ventricular [enlargement] hypertrophy. During the course of the study nine out of ten Altace® patients did not develop left ventricular enlargement. If left ventricle enlargement had already been present from the outset of the trial the ace inhibitor gradually reduced it."

The Journal article study authors claimed, "The underuse of life-saving medications in patients with systolic heart failure is a pervasive problem throughout the health care community." Frederick Masoudi, M.D., M.S.P.H., an assistant professor of medicine at Denver Health Center and the University of Colorado at Denver and lead author of the study said, "Our findings provide good evidence to validate current guideline recommendations that all patients with systolic dysfunction should be getting ACE inhibitors, unless they have a contraindication to the use of these drugs." Compiled data from the Centers from the National Heart Care Project show that 32% of elderly heart failure patients left the hospital without being given prescriptions for ACE inhibitors. "Patients discharged without anti-angiotensin therapy had a 14% greater risk of dying within a year compared to patients treated with ACE inhibitors."

Other Ways ACE Inhibitors Help Extend Life

Remipril, (Altace®) has proven to be one of those drugs providing added benefits for heart failure patients in connection with modifying high blood pressure values. This drug has proven concurrently to provide remarkable advantage against other ailments including diabetic neuropathy. The medical profession took a real serious look at Altace® when a January 2000 edition of the *New England Journal of Medicine* first reported remarkable statistics. As Altace® was proving itself effective for what it was originally intended [a blood pressure medicine] it also dramatically reduced death from all causes by 16%!

When the placebo group was compared to the Altace group, the Altace® group had exhibited a 25% less chance of dying from any cardiovascular event compared to the placebo group. Further, the members of the Altace group proved to be 20% less likely to experience a heart attack. The study also concluded that this group was 31% less likely to suffer a stroke than the placebo group. The reported benefits do not end here, as there was also a 37% reduction in sudden death cases from rhythm disturbance as determined by the SOLD study. (Study of Left

Ventricle Dysfunction). There was a 16% reduction in a need to have angioplasty or bypass surgeries among the Altace® study participants. Those patients who have been diagnosed with peripheral vascular disease (PAD) and those presenting with coronary artery disease (CAD), heart failure, diabetes, and/or related diabetic neuropathy, might want to confer with their doctor as to whether this drug class would provide additional benefit for their particular condition and overall chances of survival particularly when the study in 2006 further validates the earlier studies.

A Valuable Ally for Diabetes Patients

Data from the HOPE (*Heart Outcomes Prevention Evaluation*) trial indicated a significant 25 to 30% reduction in the risk of death from cardiovascular disease among diabetics. Diabetes and heart disease within the same patient is a combination difficult to treat; however, these study findings should be welcomed news. Coming out of the 2001 annual sessions of The American Heart Association, was information that the ACE Inhibitors have shown an ability to control inflammation factors and offers yet another explanation as to how this class of drug might contribute to the reduction of heart attacks. Blood pressure control may actually prove to be the least of the benefits. Two minor drawbacks of the ACE inhibitors is that some patients develop an annoying chest cough and another is a negative response among some heart failure patients taking an ACE inhibitor drug and aspirin. Independent studies have suggested that pulmonary activity among these particular patients may suffer as a result of the combination. Clinical tests have also indicated that aspirin may (among certain HF patients) disturb pulmonary activity related to gas exchange, general exercise, peak exercise and oxygen uptake levels.

The amount of ASA taken daily during the study was 325 mgs. How smaller amounts of daily ASA would affect these exercise and pulmonary outcomes was not determined in the particular study. A doctor will evaluate and determine on a case-by-case basis whether or not the benefits outweigh the risk of taking aspirin with each individual patient. I think you will agree these are absolutely outstanding statistics in favor of ACE inhibitor drugs. There are many drugs on the market that fall into the Ace Inhibitor class as those listed below but it was Altace that produced the findings we have just reviewed.

- Accupril
- Aceon
- Altace
- Capoten
- Lotensin
- Mavik
- Monopril
- Prinivil
- Univasc
- Vasotec
- Zestril

CHAPTER 22

What's up with the *Downside* of *Cholesterol* and *Statin Drugs?*

tudies link very low cholesterol to the following partial list of associated dysfunctions

• Hostile, aggressive, violent behavior and depression.

• Coenzyme Q10 Deficiency and A Weakened Heart
Muscle.

• Permanent Nerve and Muscle Damage.

• Loss of Memory.

• Increased Risk of Hemorrhagic stroke.

It is after all hyperlipidinemia (lipid dysfunction) which
develops into coronary artery disease. It is coronary artery
disease that leads to heart attacks, the primary link to congestive heart failure and subsequently finally creating the
need for stem cell repair. Because cholesterol and statins

remain the most talked about health issue in America, the following groundbreaking information about statins and their side effects belongs in this presentation. The fact had crossed my mind that not many people are going to want to hear something negative or even cautionary about a therapy that is in many cases life saving. After all, what could possibly be dangerous about lowering cholesterol? Let me make the point very clearly so that the information you are about to read is not misconstrued. There is no question (as the recent studies have shown) that even lowered LDL levels than has been previously suggested is better. Therefore, lowering LDL cholesterol is not the issue. How low total cholesterol (TC) must drop to attain the LDL target goal is. My job as the author is to bring you the information and your job (if I may presume) will be to decipher and use what you will from the studies and sources presented. What you are going to hear about is revolutionary and in possibly in several ways, alarming. If you are wondering if this information is designed to encourage you to stop statin therapy, it is not, unless you experience the symptoms outlined within the piece. Ultimately your doctor will be your best arbiter as to whether you continue, discontinue or reduce your current drug dosage

The Government Statin Side Effect Study

The University of California at San Diego (UCSD), along with the NIH (National Institute of Health) is currently conducting The Statin Side Effect Study to better determine the scope of the problem among patients. While the medical industry insists that only 2-3% of patients using statins report muscle aches and cramping, the UCSD study is finding otherwise. Meet M.D., Ph.D., Beatrice Golomb the study's Principal Investigational Officer who will be our guide through this cholesterol statin drug maze. Dr. Golomb is ultimately qualified to do this. I feel compelled to list her career highlights because, what she is about to discuss with us regarding statin side effects will be new to most of us, indeed even to her profession. Her training in physics and medicine, Ph.D., in neurobiology at UCSD, MD from UCSD, Chief Resident in internal medicine at the VA (Veterans Administration) in West LA and a fellowship in epidemiology/health services research with RAND/UCLA (Rand Corporation). Dr. Golomb has dedicated years to this research of statin side effects and is recognized for her scholarship and authority worldwide. She was kind enough to render an unlimited amount of time for my interview.

Dr. Golomb began by explaining that very often patients represent to the study coordinators that their physicians have failed to associate with statin therapy their complaints of memory loss, impaired cognitive function, fatigue, headaches, muscle and nerve aches, erectile dysfunction, skin rash and gastrointestinal, psychiatric or neurological problems. Dr. Golomb suggests, "There is a very simple way to prove or disprove the connection. Many of the patient's symptoms cease when they discontinue taking the drug only to have them re-appear, once they go back on therapy." She also explains, "98% of patients [complaints] taking Lipitor® (astorvastatin) and one-third of the patients taking lovastatin (Mevacor®) suffer from significant and sometimes permanent muscle problems." She has identified the damage as myopathy (myocitis) and polyneuropathy (polymyocitis). Very importantly, she explained, "The longer the individual is on a statin, the greater the risk of developing long term side affects." These side effects, according to the doctor, can be serious, multiple, complex, debillitating and sometimes fatal. These findings support those of the NIH/UCSD study."

A Non-inflammatory Form of Myopathy

The dominant complaint Dr. Golumb hears concerns a phenomenon called "non-CK (creatine kinase) elevating myopathies." She explains, "While inflammatory myopathies do certainly occur and blood tests might indicate a warning to the physician, this new form of myopathy does not. Therefore, without the dysfunction identified, the undetected muscle and nerve damage may continue until the it possibly becomes irreversible." The UCSD findings of non-inflammatory myopathy were also reaffirmed by a presentation to an American Medical Association Conference in 2002 by Dr. Paul Phillips of Scripps Mercy Hospital in San Diego, CA. Dr. Phillips reported that many statin patients were experiencing very painful side effects even though their blood tests did not show elevations in CK. These findings support those of the NIH/UCSD study.

Greater Risk with Longer Statin Use

Dr. Golomb has pointed out, "The side effects become more and more obvious the longer an individual is on the drug." Note: Physicians normally monitor a patient during the first 3-6 months of statin use. Test results in the short term may indicate the drug is being well tolerated and therefore there is no need to test patients again for another two, three or even five years. The physician, unaware of the information the study's principal investigator shares with us, may not make a connection between statins and the muscle, nerve and cognitive symptoms a patient may be experiencing, particularly when these symptoms can quite easily be explained away as arthritis, rheumatism, gout or any one of more than 100 ailments. Clouding the issue for the physician is the information pharmaceutical companies and their representatives bring to doctors' offices, insisting that statin side effects are absolutely minimal.

The 500,000-person Danish Gaist study published in the journal *Neurology* May 2000 found that a significant 15% of patients, reportedly developed nerve damage after taking a statin, for just one year. Damage was reported as progressive and rose even more dramatically to an alarming 26% during the second year of the patient's therapy! The increase in symptoms, according to the study findings, would affect one in four patients and the 26% increase is obviously more than the 1-2 or even 3% rate of patient complaints drug companies have been admitting to.

"Statin Side Effects are Dose Related, Some Patients May Never Recover"—Golomb

Director Golomb has determined, "the degree of risks for side effects are found to be dose related," as she has said. "The higher the prescription dosage the greater the number and severity of the complaints." She offered the following scenario, "Patients whose muscle symptoms precipitated from statin use may never completely recover and the myopathy may not in all cases be completely reversed." Dr. Golomb continued, "It is difficult to extrapolate accurate myopathy numbers from the studies because many trials only define myopathy as detrimental when the CK levels exceed 10 times the upper limit of normal and is accompanied by sore muscle adverse affects." At this point of advancing muscle or nerve damage in a patient's history Dr. Golomb added, "it would be acknowledged that the patient might already suffer from advanced rabdomyolysis (rab-do-my-äl-i-sis) kidney failure or even death. "Those affected patients who are disabled and discomforted by an impaired ability to walk and are suffering severe pain from myopathy caused by a statin drug, could care less whether or not their CK level has reached the 10 times above normal level, that would alarm their physicians. They have already reached crisis in their daily lives and in many cases that crisis is being overlooked because the CK level (by current testing) appears normal or only slightly elevated. Even if patients are not technically diagnosed with rabdomyolysis, they already have a significant compromise in quality of life and inability to exercise and they, therefore, miss all of the benefits and protection exercise would afford."

If the San Diego study is finding myopathy present in patients who do not present with significantly or even modestly elevated CK levels then it would appear that something is being overlooked in the present risk assessment. That very oversight would be extending the element of undetected serious risk to certain patients and possibly even to you and me. It was apparent, as evidenced by the thousands of filed patient complaints registered with the San Diego study group as well as those listed on the Lipitor®, AARP, RXlist and government drug complaint websites, that the issue of drug side effects and the statin link needed to be explored. The UCSD study is designed to fulfill that need—not only by evaluating the full set of muscle effects but considering other manifestations and complications as well, including memory loss, (loss of) cognitive function, fatigue, tendonitis, malaise and depression.

A Two Edged Sword

There is absolutely no argument as to the definite benefits from statin drugs in slowing the development of heart disease. Several studies, including the (Scandinavian Simvastatin Survival Study) have shown that statins do interfere with the development and advancement of coronary artery disease. Nonetheless, as the UCSD study demonstrates, there is a growing body of evidence suggesting that statins in all their glory and benefit also pose serious side effects for tens of thousands of patients. Certainly, if we are exchanging one set of health problems for another, the trade off must be examined.

Lessons from Another Dose Related Case

The FDA's own Director of Science David J. Graham, standing before the US Senate hearing in the Merck/Vioxx case, emphasized a dose related increase in risk as follows: a low dose of Vioxx brought a 50% heart disease increase while in comparison the high dose brought the risk up 358%. Clearly, Dr. Graham was not talking about statin therapy at this point in his presentation but the message to take from his testimony is that dosage drug levels do make a difference.

Dosage amount suddenly take on a whole new meaning as physicians have recently been advised to double or even triple statin strength to achieve more optimal LDL goals. Incidentally, during Graham's appearance before the US Senate, he did actually take the opportunity to voice his concern over the statin drug Crestor® (rosuvastatin). "When Crestor® was submitted in its higher dose version to the government for approval," said Graham, "the application was denied." What does this denial tell us about dose related risk side effects? According to the FDA some 20 million people and 150 million around the world are currently taking statin drugs to ameliorate their risk of heart attacks and strokes. Now that the newest studies suggest seeking a much-lowered LDL range (66-70) for hi-risk heart patients, another 30 million people may now fall under the category of statin patients. If Dr. Golomb and the other researchers who have been studying this problem for many years are correct in their claims, there will be an even greater number of side effects reported as the new recommended increased dosages are generally assimilated by statin drug users.

So present and in our face are the pharmaceutical sales and marketing campaigns that we patients are actually doing the manufacturers' sales job for them. We see their commercials 24/7 and end up asking our doctors to put us on a particular medication we saw advertised. Don't most of the commercials end with the phrase, "Talk to your doctor?" This statement is followed by the disclaimer that such and such a drug may not be right for everyone, serious side effects may occur in some cases. The drug companies have cleverly taken their sales pitch to the public to enlist us as part of their sales team in their constant need and desire to sell their drugs. This is a $4.5 billion industry and the ads are cleverly designed to solicit our help in convincing our doctors to do the drug company's job for them. What a boon to the statin drug manufacturers the newest recommended guidelines have brought, urging higher dosage and qualifying another 30 million prospective statin users. A bill has been introduced by Senator Ron Wyden of (Oregon) and quoted in the LA Times article in June 2005 titled, Wary and Weary of Drug Ads, the bill's author said, "They [drug companies] make a lot more if patients without medical degrees are encouraged to start writing their own prescriptions, whether the drug is the right one or not." Wyden is not the only legislator calling for stronger controls and guidelines for drug companies. James Moran (Rep. Va) is going after the erectile dysfunction drug advertisers.

If there ever was a sales job done on the public, the four-hour enticement claim is oversell at it's best. There is an increase in the number of doctors and law makers proposing legislation for tighter controls on the drug sales to the public approach, perceived as a practice that is driving drug costs even higher as more and more patients demand drugs that they might not really need. One physician admitted he gave in to his patients' requests 45% of the time. If they didn't get the prescription from me, he said, they would get it somewhere else. There is another issue and that is doctors only have so much valuable time with patients to discuss their serious medical conditions. An interesting article appeared in a June 2005 edition of USA Today by Robert Centor titled, "Take Drug Ads Off The Air," Centor was addressing this very same issue.

"In an ideal world, the physician could take all the time necessary to explain why the drug [advertised] isn't right for that particular patient. Discussing these requests causes two problems: a) other important issues are set aside, and b) physicians must decide whether to have a lengthy discussion or take the course of least resistance, acceding to the insistent requests."

Natural Alternatives for Patients Who Cannot Tolerate Statins?

More and more physicians are looking to non-statin choices, with an interest in helping their patients who are unable to assimilate statin drugs. Among the pack of possible substitutes from the plant sterol class is policosonal, made from sugar cane. Other plant versions being sold, as policosonal are not as effective as the product derived from sugar cane. Having gone through multiple controlled studies, policosonal (PAC) (Polyenylphosphatidylchloride) is reportedly considered safe with almost zero side effects. The efficacy of policosonal in a study by (Castano et al. Prat 1999) compared favorably to three of the popular HMG CoA inhibitor (statin) drugs. Policosonal of 10 mgs a day given to (55 patients) was compared to lovastatin (Mevacor®) 20 mg/day given to (26 patients) and simvastatin (Zocor®) of 10 mg/day given to (25 patients), the following results were reported at the end of 6 weeks:

LDL comparisons

• 24% reduction in LDL with policosonal.

• 22% reduction with lovastatin.

• 15% reduction with simvastatin.

Policosonal study subjects had improved LDL to HDL

ratios between 17.2% and 26.5%, along with a 7% increased benefit in total HDL. There was also an improved lowering benefit to blood pressure. Another natural substitute, guggul/gugulipid (made from the sap of the mukul tree) has also shown remarkable results as an alternative substitute to statins as evidenced by one of several reported studies: According to (Agarwal, 1986; Nityanand 1989) guggul brought a lipid improvement in 70% of study subjects with an LDL improvement of between 14-27% and HDL was also reported improved among 60% of patients. The natural plant sterol beta-sistosterol and Chinese red yeast are both very effective in lowering cholesterol but it should be noted that red yeast is what the first statin drug was made from and should be monitored with liver tests, as with any other statin. A proven natural cholesterol reducer that can often drop the level 20% is the popular breakfast cereal, oatmeal. Niacin is also an effective substitute but because of potential (passive but annoying) side effects such as tingling and flushing of the skin if taken in too great an amount at the outset of therapy. The effect can be eliminated in one of several ways. Taking slow-release timed release niacin or the instant release form but in very small doses taken with food and increased gradually to tolerance. An aspirin an hour before also helps eliminate the flush. Physicians often prescribe niacin in the prescription Niaspan® that can be given in high dosage without the tingling or facial flushing side effects. There is one abiding fact when it comes to taking any drug: With every drug you take to solve one dysfunction another dysfunction is often created. [Policonsonal may not be as effective for patients with a genetic lipid dysfunction ed. Note]

Cause and Effect with Taking Drugs

Here are listed just a few examples of how one drug can replace one problem with another. As effective as niacin is (hundreds of thousands take it) to raise good HDL cholesterol and lower triglycerides, it will independently raise homocysteine 50%! Homocysteine, when elevated is recognized as a two to three fold contributor to cardiovascular and stroke disease. The popular fibrate drug fenofibrate (Tricor®), while offering excellent HDL and triglyceride results, has also been reported in a study to also raise homocysteine 41%. Fibrinogen, recognized in the Framingham Heart Study and by the American Heart Association as an independent risk factor for heart attack and stroke will reportedly increase 20% when one is taking Lipitor® (40 mgs), and as well rises 20% when taking the fibrate drug gemfibrozil. (ATVB 1995: Adriana Branchi) Seldom are fibrinogen levels checked. The health conscious public was surprised to learn suddenly that drinking grapefruit juice or eating the fruit itself would negate or minimize the effects of a statin drug. For every action there is a reaction; for every drug taken for one advantage, another disadvantage is created. Sometimes it seems you just can't win for losing.

Statins Lower Inflammation

It is now an established fact that statin drugs perform a dual role in both lowering inflammation and controlling bad cholesterol. A widely held opinion among leading cardiologists is that the anti-inflammatory effect is even more the reason why statins have lowered the death rate from heart disease. One might make the argument that a patient experiencing severe statin side effects would lose the anti-inflammatory benefit of the statin if it became necessary to replace the drug with one of the alternative non-statin therapies. Natural inflammatory fighters that have consistently proven effective in lowering inflammation include the following:

1. Turmeric (curcuma longa), an herb used in preparation of curry dishes and also known as curcurmin, is considered one of the most effective natural anti-inflammatory sources.

2. Bromelain, an enzyme derived from pineapple besides aiding in better digestion in the breakdown of food also provides anti-inflammatory properties.

3. Aspirin (ASA), a third inflammatory fighter, happens to be an age-old remedy. Aspirin, as mentioned in an earlier chapter, was found in the landmark government Physician's Health Study to lower inflammation 55.7%.

All of these alternative non-statin choices should be discussed with your physician, particularly if you are experiencing muscle aches and pains. Some physicians, acknowledging as has Dr. Golomb, that the side effects from statins are dose related may even choose to prescribe a lower dose statin but to fortify the regimen with one of the natural alternatives.

Cholesterol Too Low?

I had an interesting discussion with a doctor friend two years ago who kept asking me to guess his cholesterol. I said, no, I don't think I want to guess. Suppose you tell me. I know you're dying to anyway. He looked like he was about to share the word's biggest secret. "My cholesterol," he half whispered, "is 111!" Are you nuts came my reply? Are you not aware of the almost two dozen studies that show the multiple dangers when total cholesterol drops that low? What about the increased risk of stroke?

My friend got up from his desk invited me to sit at his computer and said, "Show me." I searched out a French study that had first appeared in the *British Medical Journal* in mid 1996, reporting on a study that had 6,390 male participants. The study parameters were concentrated on death by suicide and found that men with the lowest cholesterol levels [because of inadequate seratonin] were 3 times more likely to take their own lives than those with higher cholesterol levels. I recognize that one study does not establish a medical fact and because I was talking to a man of science, I was determined to find at least two studies supportive of my claim before I left his office. I located a second study in the *American Journal of Psychiatry* that had been published in the first quarter of 1995. This particular study had divided the participants into four categories, from the lowest cholesterol level to the highest. The study's authors determined that those men in the lower ranges were twice as likely to commit suicide as those in the higher ranges.

So there is no misunderstanding, we are continuing to talk about the total cholesterol level and not the LDL. There is no argument, the lower the LDL the better. So the second issue becomes, "How does one lower the bad LDL cholesterol to 60-70-85 mg/dl without dropping the overall total cholesterol into life threatening territory?" Two other points need to be considered. One is that low cholesterol among seniors is very worrisome and numerous studies have established a level of 180 to 200 mg/dl to be supportive for longevity. The second consideration is whether dropping total cholesterol levels among seniors to 140-130 120 mg/dl is in the best interest in prolonging the lives of seniors? To better understand the risks the following stroke information is offered.

CHAPTER 23

Stroke: *the* Number 3 Killer

S troke ranks behind heart disease and cancer as the number three killer of Americans, It also has the undesirable distinction of being the number one disabler of American adults. 700,000 people in a given year in America experience a stroke, which result in a 160,000 deaths. When we become aware that an astounding number of 140, 938 of the deaths occur among patients 65 or older we have to ask "Is the link between cholesterol and stroke being fully realized for the elderly patient?" To put that huge number of deaths in perspective, comparatively speaking, there are only 3,418 patients who die in any given year under the age of 44. If studies have established the level of 180-200 mg/dl as better contributing to longevity among the elderly and levels below 180 as producing more fatal strokes among the same group, what should be a safe accepted protocol protective to seniors? According to the evidence just presented, a mistake in over prescribing lowering medication could have grave consequence.

Low Cholesterol and Greater Risk of Hemorrhagic Stroke

A presentation at the American Heart Association's 24th annual Conference on Stroke and Cerebral Circulation by Dr. David Tirschwell of the University of Washington. The reported information claimed that a greater risk for hemorrhagic stroke existed when the total cholesterol level was lower than 180 mgs and confirmed a two-fold augmented stroke risk compared to someone with a reading of 230 mgs. As explained by Dr. Tirshwell, very low cholesterol could compromise the integrity of the vessel walls within the brain allowing blood to literally seep through the brain's membrane. [Ed note], This membrane breakdown is in fact, an accurate description of a hemorrhagic stroke. How then can aggressively lowering total cholesterol to achieve an ideal LDL level be acceptable if it controls cholesterol at the risk of exposing an elderly patient to serious stroke risk? The safe level ascertained in the various studies for senior patients is between 180-200 mg/dl.

Understanding the Kinds of Stroke Hemorrhagic Stroke

While only accounting for 20% of all the stroke cases in America, this form of stroke carries a staggering fatality rate of between 45 and 50%. There is a significant 40-

80% death rate during the 30-day period immediately following a hemorrhagic stroke. This is the form of stroke that befell Israel's Ariel Sharon in 2006 leaving him in a vegetative state even after multiple surgeries to ameliorate the damage caused by the stroke. As if these statistics are not discouraging enough, half the deaths from hemorrhagic stroke will occur within the first 48 hours. We have not talked about aneurysms but they are associated with hemorrhagic strokes. Another stroke fact is that African Americans fall victim to a disproportionate number of both kinds of strokes and statistically, 71% of all black women will die as a consequence of stroke.

Ischemic Stroke

The ischemic stroke is the most common form of stroke that accounts for 88% of all strokes (according to the American Heart Association). It is the stroke whose damage we are quick to recognize as it manifests in physical deformity, facial paralysis, slurred speech or a limp arm or leg. It also can affect mental function and motor skills. The causes are most often uncontrolled high blood pressure and/or a history of elevated cholesterol that has formed deposits within the arteries and vessels that either grow to occlude an artery or dislodge plaque from a vessel wall to block blood flow to the brain itself. Particularly vulnerable are clots in the carotid arteries. Fifty percent of the stroke victims will survive the initial attack but another 25% will not survive and the remaining 25%% will experience long-term disabilities dealing daily with moderate to very severe health problems. So on one hand there is the danger from one form of stroke (ischemic) caused by high cholesterol deposits, while on the other hand the second form (hemorrhagic) is caused by the opposite phenomena of cholesterol actually being too low.

TIA (Transient Ischemic Attack)

TIA, as its name implies, is a transient attack and symptoms will usually pass. The American Heart Association cautions that TIA should be considered a warning of a more serious impending stroke. Symptoms from a TIA may be slurred speech, partial loss of vision (possibly in one eye) and disorientation. A Doppler ultrasound will usually be ordered by the physician in order to rule out obstruction or narrowing in the carotid arteries.

Embolic Stroke (embolus)

An embolism can form on the wall of an artery, become dislodged and circulate through the blood stream as a clot or air bubble. It can form somewhere outside the brain but eventually moves to block a vessel within the brain. In the case of a pulmonary embolism the clot migrates from the leg to the lung.

Thrombotic Stroke

A thrombus is a circulating emboli that forms a permanent clot attaching itself to a vessel wall. A thrombosis commonly forms within an artery, within a chamber of the heart, or forms within the brain creating a cerebral thrombotic stroke. Controlling blood pressure, LDL cholesterol and monitoring clotting factors are all important to minimize the risks associated with having a stroke.

Aspirin (ASA) and Stroke

The Journal *Stroke* in 1999 published a study that confirmed while low dose aspirin was helpful in preventing an ischemic stroke too much aspirin could actually bring about a hemorrhagic stroke.

Low Cholesterol Linked to Hostile Aggressive, Violent Behavior, Depression and Suicide

Side effects from low cholesterol have been reported in studies besides nerve and muscle damage also include depression. The link between statin drugs and depression has been very well established and the reasons are plausible, understandable and medically logical when one views the literature regarding low cholesterol and seratonin levels. The connection becomes more of a concern when newer guidelines suggest accepting even lower cholesterol levels if one has familial history of premature heart disease, hypertension or for those who smoke. In order to do so, the doctor and the patient agree to double or even triple the daily dosage of their statin. Stockholders in companies like Phizer, who makes Lipitor® (astorvastatin), Merck, who makes both lovastatin (Mevacor®) and simavastin (Zocor®) and Astrazeneca the manufacturer of rosuvastatin (Crestor®) are ecstatic. Total cholesterol is dropping and corporate incomes are rising accordingly. The patient and his/her doctor (not all doctors of course) are thrilled at seeing readings of total cholesterol in the 140-120 or even 110 ranges. There is absolutely no argument (as has been the contention) that a lowered LDL is an ideal and attainable goal. The question is "At what price and where do you draw the line on the side of caution in how much you can afford to drop the total cholesterol?" It is worth noting that, as the doctor gives the patient advice to control his/her cholesterol, the patient is also advised to watch his/her diet, monitor saturated fat intake and engage in more exercise. All proven, solid and excellent advice. These elements by themselves might have brought the cholesterol into acceptable ratios but with increased dosage consider how low the total cholesterol could be following 60-90 days of therapy.

Low Cholesterol and Violent Behavior, is it all in the Head?

Dr. Golomb's report done at UCLA (Low Serum Cholesterol and Violent Behavior) in 1998 examined a link between low cholesterol and violence as documented in journal articles dating back to 1965. One study in particular had recorded an obvious upsurge in violent behavior in monkeys when their cholesterol became low.

Other randomized trials found excess violent deaths among men who were administered statin therapy even though they were not heart patients and did not require it. Researcher Marc Hillbrand [et al] had found in studying violent behavior among 25 psychiatric patients, "total serum cholesterol concentration was positively associated with measures that affect cognitive efficiency, activation, and sociability, suggesting a link between low total serum cholesterol and [negative presence of mind]." That would appear a pretty strong indictment against dropping total cholesterol too low.

Statin and Fibrate Drugs Together

"We found," says Dr. Golomb, "Gemfribrozil [a widely prescribed fibrate] blocks two vital metabolic pathways creating a significant amount of rabdomyolysis and fenofibrate (Tricor®), a second fibrate drug, comparatively blocked one metabolic pathway when taken with a statin." The information suggests one is courting an invitation to trouble when a fibrate and statin are administered in combination even though the practice would seem logically to make sense. While the fibrate drug successfully raises the HDL and lowers the triglycerides it will not have the same effect on LDL and total cholesterol. The approach of taking a statin along with a fibrate might well attain the proposed objective but possibly at a greater price than one would want to pay. The cautionary warnings were there in prescribing Vioxx®, Bextra® and

Celebrex® but the positive effects were so impressive and the patient need for relief so profound that it was felt the benefit outweighed the risk. Should we learn from what has transpired and not make the same mistake with the statin/fibrate combination?

We have been on an informative journey together that began at the very first chapter titled: *The Possible Impossible Dream*. It should now be obvious that we, as a society, stand on the brink of amazing medical breakthroughs in the treatment of catastrophic disease. It is also apparent that indeed, the impossible is not only possible, but also inevitable. It is a good time to be living. My hope for you and your family is that you never need intervention, but if you do, that the technology and science is ready and available.

Sincerely yours,

Christian Wilde

Appendix I Glossary

ACE inhibitors, an angiotensis blood pressure medication with additional benefits.

Alzheimers, a disease robbing the elderly of mental function.

Allogenic, transplanting from one to another or in the same patient.

Anaphylactic shock, causing life threatening drops in blood pressure.

Aneurysm, a bulge within a heart or brain artery.

Angina Pectoris, "heart pain", from blood and oxygen starvation.

Angiogenesis, growing of natural bypass vessels around blockages.

Angiogram, permits visualization of arterial interiors.

Angiography, science and technology study within arteries.

Angioplasty, a procedure that opens an obstructed artery by balloon inflation.

Antioxidants, which fight oxidation.

Aortic valve, main heart valve located in the aorta.

Arrhythmia, irregular heartbeat.

Arterioles, tiny vessels that grow to permit blood around a blockage.

Arteriosclerosis,thickening, hardening of the arterial walls, loss of elasticity.

Asymptomatic, not showing symptoms.

Atheroma, fatty degeneration on the inner arterial wall.

Atherosclerosis, cholesterol and fatty deposit buildup in the coronary arteries.

Autologous, donor and recipient are same person.

Atrial fibrillation, atrium beating out of control and rhythm with the rest of the heart.

Atrium, upper heart chamber receiving blood from the veins sending it to the ventricles.

Baycol, a discontinued statin drug linked to many deaths.

Beta Blockers, a class of drug that slows the heart's beat and work load.

Beta-carotene, antioxidant containing vitamin A.

Blastocyst, formed of pluripotent cells that form the developing embryo.

Brain attack, a mini (TIA), or major stroke..

Bruit, a blockage in a carotid artery heard by stethoscope.

By-pass, a surgery replacing diseased coronary arteries with leg or mammary arteries.

Calcification, deposits of calcium into tissues or heart valves.

Cardiologists, medical doctors specializing in care of the cardiovascular system.

Cardiomyopathy, chronic damaged heart muscle from disease or enlargement.

Cardio-thoracic surgeon, operates on the heart and lungs.

Carotid arteries, the arteries in the neck leading to the brain.

Chlamydia pneumoniae, a bacterial disease caused by upper respiratory illness.

Chlamydia pneumoniae, a bacterial infection causing upper respiratory illness.

CMV, cytomegaliovirus, a viral infection involved with heart disease.

Coenzyme Q10, required by every cell in the body, vital to heart muscle.

Cognitive function, elements of mental function.

Collateral arteries, small formed naturally around a blockage.

Collateral vessels, another name for "natural bypass."

Congestive Heart Failure, an inefficient functioning heart.

CPR, Cardio pulmonary resuscitation.

C-reactive protein, a marker of bodily inflammation.

CRP, C-reactive protein, an acute phase reactant marker of inflammation.

CT, ultrasound computerized tomography.

Defibrillator, a device that shocks the heart back into rhythm.

Diabetes Mellitus, a vascular disorder of carbohydrate metabolism, a vascular disease.

Diagnostic, test to determine illness or wellness.

Diuretics, promote urination of fluid and salts.

Doppler ultrasound, a technology using sound waves to measure obstruction.

Drug resistant, a disease that has built an immunity to available medication.

DVT, deep vein thrombosis, clots formed within the legs and recesses of the calf.

Dysfunction, not functioning as normal.

Dyslipidemia, out of control cholesterol level.

Echocardiogram, uses sound waves to observe shapes and certain organ functions.

ECP, Enhanced counterpulsation.

ECG, electrocardiogram.

EKG, measures electric activity.

Edema, accumulation of fluid in blood vessels in legs and abdomen.

EECP®, Trademarked, Enhanced External Counterpulsation.

EF, ejection fraction, measurement of heart functionability.

Ejection fraction, the measurement of how the blood is forced from the heart to the body.

EKG, electrocardiogram, a machine that records the electrical function of the heart.

Embolic, as related to an embolism.

Embolism, a sudden obstruction of clot formation.

Embolus, a particle that circulates in the blood.

Embryo, an animal in the early stages of growth and dif-ferentiation.

Embryonic, a being in the early stage of development.

EMT, Emergency medical treatment.

Endarterectomy, serious surgery to open carotid blockage.

Endothelium, fine smooth linings of the arteries.

ER, emergency room.

Fibrates, a form of cholesterol drug most effective for triglyceride and HDL dysfunction.

Fibrillation, beating out of sync and rhythm.

Fibrin, formed from fibrinogen in clot formation.

Fibrinogen, a blood protein involved in stroke, plaque and heart disease.

Folic acid, of the B complex family, folate.

Framingham Study, early government heart study.

Genomics, study of the structure of the genome of particular organisms.

H. pylori, a bacterial infection suspect in heart disease.

Hardening of the arteries, arteriosclerosis.

HCM, (hypertrophic cardiomyopathy).

HDL, high density lipoprotein (good cholesterol).

Helicobactor Pylori, a bacterial infection affecting heart disease.

Homogenous, familiar, compatible.

Hemorrhagic, prone to excessive bleeding, a form of stroke.

HMO, health managed organization.

Homocysteine, a sulphur containing byproduct of methionine.

Homocysteininemia, high (HCY) possibly heredity related.

H-Pylori, abbreviation for helicobacter pylori, an infection associated with ulcers.

Hypertension, high blood pressure.

Hypertrophic cardiomyopathy (HCM), thickening of heart walls.

IABP, intra-aortic balloon pump.

ICU, Intensive care unit.

Inflammatory markers, blood tests that record inflammation.

Inherited, a risk factor of genetic origin.

Insulin, a hormone produced by the pancreas involved with diabetes.

Interventional cardiologists, cardiologists who perform procedures inside the arteries.

Ischemia, a reduction in normal flow of the blood to the heart.

IVUS, intravascular ultrasound.

JAMA, journal of the American Heart Association.

LDL, low density lipoprotein (bad).

Left main artery, where most major heart attacks strike.

Lineage, varieties, continuing lines.

Lumen, the open area within an artery.

LVAD, left-ventricle assist device aiding function of left ventricle.

Mesenchymal, versatile bone marrow cells.

Macular degeneration, leading cause of blindness among seniors.

Metabolic process, affected by metabolism.

Mevacor, (lovastatin) the first statin drug.

Microscopy, examination by microscope.

Minimally invasive, opening only the smallest area necessary during surgery.

Molecular, relating to, or consisting of molecules.

Multipotent, cell types found to behave like neurons or brain cells.

Multi-vessel heart disease, occurring within more than one artery.

Myoblast, A primitive muscle cell having the potential to develop into a muscle fiber.

Natural by-pass, body's ability to grow smaller vessels around a blockage.

Niacin, vitamin B3, also known as nicotinic acid and the trade name niaspan.

Niaspan, a prescribed form of time release niacin.

Non-invasive, procedures that do not enter the body.

Novel, uncommon.

Nuclear treadmill, utilizes a liquid agent to trace blood flow to all areas of the heart.

Occlusion, blockage in an artery .

Olfactory stem cells, found in the olfactory sciences.

Omega 3, an important oil beneficial against heart attack and stroke.

PAD, (peripheral artery disease).

Paraplegia, paralysis affecting the legs.

Pathologist, whose science deals with tissues.

Peripheral artery disease, (PAD) heart disease extended beyond the coronary arteries.

Plaque, the buildup of fat deposits, fibrin, calcium within the arteries or vessels.

Platelet aggregation, sticking of platelets together.

Pluripotent, a pluripotent cell is one able to differentiate into most cell types.

Polyunsaturated fat, a good fat.

Postmortem, after death.

Predisposition, prone to as in family inherited traits.

Prenisone, a popular steroid.

Prognosis, what is medically expected.

Prophylaxis, a preventive.

Proteomics, the study of all the proteins that make up an organism.

Pulmonary embolism, a blood clot in the lung or lung artery.

Quadipilegia, paralysis affecting the arms and legs.

Regimen, a planned therapy.

Regimen, a pre-set routine.

Regurgitating blood, blood flow rejected by a diseased heart valve.

Re-stenosis, a repeated obstruction or blockage.

Saturated, undesirable fats from animal sources.

Silent heart attack, occurring without symptoms or without knowledge.

Silent ischemia, diminished blood flow not obvious symptomatically to the patient.

Silent stroke, one occurring to areas of the brain that do not show symptoms.

Sleep apnea, a sleep condition where the breathing stops due to obstructed airway.

Staph infection, staphylococcus aureus contracted through an open incision.

Stenosis, obstruction or blockage.

Stents, small metal sleeves inserted into an artery to keep it open.

Syndrome X, an endangering combination of factors in diabetes.

Testicular, stem cells extracted from the testes.

Thallium treadmill, utilizes a tracing agent to follow blood flow throughout the heart.

Thrombosis, resulting from development and collection

of a clot within an artery.

Thrombus, a stationary clot clinging to its point of origin.

TIA, (temporary ischemic attack), a mini stroke, precursor of major stroke.

Totipotent, cells that can develop to any tissue.

Trans fats, dangerous form of processed fat.

Triglycerides, made from stored sugars and fats circulating in the blood.

Ultra-fast CT, a CT scan that captures pictures between heart beats.

Unstable plaque, ready to dislodge at anytime.

Vascular diseases, affecting the heart arteries and vascular system.

Ventricle fibrillation, the ventricle flutters out of time.

Ventricle, receives blood from the upper atrium, sends to the body.

Vioxx®, a discontinued arthritis drug linked to many deaths.

Viscosity, thickness of the blood.

Vulnerable Plaque, plaque most prone to rupture from an artery wall.

WBC, (White Cell Count).

"Widow maker," dubious title for the LAD (left Anterior Descending) artery.

Appendix II References

Skeletal Myoblasts

1. **Taylor, D.A.** (2001) *Cellular cardiomyoplasty with autologous skeletal myoblasts for ischemic heart disease and heart failure.* Curr Control Trials Cardiovasc Med 2, 208-210.
2. **Taylor, D.A., Hruban, R., Rodriguez, E.R., Goldschmidt-Clermont, P.J.** *Cardiac chimerism as a mechanism for self-repair: does it happen and if so to what degree? Circulation.*
3. **Dib, N., Diethrich, E.B., Campbell, A., Goodwin, N., Robinson, B., Gilbert, J., Hobohm, D.W., Taylor, D.A.** *Endoventricular transplantation of allogenic skeletal myoblasts in a porcine model of myocardial infarction.* J Endovasc 9(3), 313-319.
4. **Van den Bos, E.J., Taylor, D.A.** *Cardiac transplantation of skeletal myoblasts for heart failure.* Minerva Cardioangiologica Apr, 51(2), 227-243.
5. **Rauscher, F.M., Goldschmidt-Clermont, P.J., Davis, B.H., Wang, T., Ramaswami, P., Pippen, A.M., Gregg, D., Annex, B.H., Chunming, D., Taylor, D.A.** *Aging, progenitor cell exhaustion and atherosclerosis. Circulation,* Jul 29, 108(4), 457-463.
6. **Thompson, R.B., Emani, S.M., Davis, B.H., van den Bos, E.J., Morimoto Y., Craig, D., Glower, D., Taylor, D.A.** *Comparison of intracardiac cell transplantation: Autologous skeletal myoblasts versus bone marrow cells. Circulation* (in press)
7. **Kessler PD, Byrne BJ.** *Myoblast cell grafting into heart muscle: cellular biology and potential applications.* Annu Rev Physiol. 1999;61:219–242.
8. **Suzuki K, Brand NJ, Smolenski RT et al.** *Development of a novel method for cell transplantation through the coronary artery. Circulation.* 2000;102:III359–III364.
9. **Atkins BZ, Hueman MT, Meuchel JM et al.** *Myogenic cell transplantation improves in vivo regional performance in infarcted rabbit myocardium.* J Heart Lung Transplant. 1999;18:1173–1180.
10. **Menasche P, Hagege AA, Scorsin M et al.** *Myoblast transplantation for heart failure. Lancet.* 2001;357:279–280.
11. **Murry CE, Wiseman RW, Schwartz SM et al.** *Skeletal myoblast transplantation for repair of myocardial necrosis.* J Clin Invest. 1996;98:2512–2523.

12. **Dorfman J, Duong M, Zibaitis A et al.** *Myocardial tissue engineering with autologous myoblast implantation.* J Thorac Cardiovasc Surg. 1998;116:744–751.

13. **Kessler PD, Byrne BJ.** *Myoblast cell grafting into heart muscle: cellular biology and potential applications.* Annu Rev Physiol. 1999;61: 219–242.

14. **Suzuki K, Brand NJ, Smolenski RT et al.** *Development of a novel method for cell transplantation through the coronary artery. Circulation.* 2000;102:III359–III364.

15. **Atkins BZ, Hueman MT, Meuchel JM et al.** *Myogenic cell transplantation improves in vivo regional performance in infarcted rabbit myocardium.* J Heart Lung Transplant. 1999;18:1173–1180.

16. **Menasche P, Hagege AA, Scorsin M et al.** *Myoblast transplantation for heart failure.* Lancet. 2001;357:279–280.

17. **Dorfman J, Duong M, Zibaitis A et al.** *Myocardial tissue engineering with autologous myoblast implantation.* J Thorac Cardiovasc Surg. 1998;116:744–751.

18. **Ghostine S, Carrion C, Souza LC et al.** *Long-term efficacy of myoblast transplantation on regional structure and function after myocardial infarction. Circulation.* 2002;106:I131–I136.

19. **Taylor DA, Atkins BZ, Hungspreugs P et al.** *Regenerating functional myocardium: improved performance after skeletal myoblast transplantation.* Nat Med. 1998;4:929.

20. **Hagege AA, Carrion C, Menasche P et al.** *Viability and differentiation of autologous skeletal myoblast grafts in ischaemic cardiomyopathy.* Lancet. 2003;361:491–492.

21. **Chiu RC, Zibaitis A, Kao RL.** *Cellular cardiomyoplasty: myocardial regeneration with satellite cell implantation.* Ann Thorac Surg. 1995;60:12–18.

22. **Reinecke H, Poppa V, Murry CE.** *Skeletal muscle stem cells do not transdifferentiate into cardiomyocytes after cardiac grafting.* J Mol Cell Cardiol. 2002;34:241–249.

23. **Schiller NB, Shah PM, Crawford M et al.** *Recommendations for quantitation of the left ventricle by two-dimensional echocardiography. American Society of Echocardiography Committee on Standards, Subcommittee on Quantitation of Two-Dimensional Echocardiograms.* J Am Soc Echocardiogr. 1989;2:358–367.

24. **Murry CE, Wiseman RW, Schwartz SM, et al.** *Skeletal myoblast transplantation for repair of myocardial necrosis.* J Clin Invest.1996; 98: 2512-2523.

25. **Graf T.** *Differentiation plasticity of hematopoietic cells.* Blood.

2002; 99: 3089–3101.

26. **Malouf NN, Coleman WB, Girsham JW, et al.** *Adult-derived stem cells from the liver become myocytes in the heart in vivo.* Am J Pathol. 2001; 158: 1929–1935.

27. **Donovan PJ, Gearhart J.** *The end of the beginning for pluripotent stem cells.* Nature. 2001; 414: 92–97.

28. **Jackson KA, Majka SM, Wulf GG, et al.** *Stem cells: a mini-review.* J Cell Biochem. 2002; (suppl 38): 1–6.

29. **Orlic D, Hill JM, Arai AE.** *Stem cells for myocardial regeneration.* Circ Res. 2002; 91: 1092–1102

30. **Gill M, Dias S, Hattori K, et al.** *Vascular trauma induces rapid but transient mobilization of VEGFR2(+)AC133(+) endothelial precursor cells.* Circ Res. 2001; 88: 167–174.

31. **Rioufol G, Finet G, Ginon I, et al.** *Multiple atherosclerotic plaque rupture in acute coronary syndrome: a three-vessel intravascular ultrasound study.* Circulation. 2002; 106: 804–808

32. **Forrester JS, Price M, Makkar R.** *Mending the broken heart.* Clin Cardiol. 2003.

33. **Li RK, Weisel RD, Mickle DA, et al.** *Autologous porcine heart cell transplantation improved heart function after a myocardial infarction.* J Thorac Cardiovasc Surg. 2000; 119: 62–68

34. **Reinecke H, Poppa V, Murry CE.** *Skeletal muscle stem cells do not transdifferentiate into cardiomyocytes after cardiac grafting.* J Mol Cell Cardiol. 2002; 34: 241–249.

35. **Torrente Y, Camirand G, Pisati F, et al.** *Identification of a putative pathway for the muscle homing of stem cells in a muscular dystrophy model.* Cell Biol. 2003; 162: 511–520.

36. **Kocher AA, Schuster MD, Szaboles MJ, et al.** *Neovascularization of ischemic myocardium by human bone-marrow-derived angioblasts prevents cardiomyocyte apoptosis, reduces remodeling and improves cardiac function.* Nat Med. 2001; 7: 430–436.

37. **Liu Y, Rao MS.** *Transdifferentiation: fact or artifact.* J Cell Biochem. 2003; 88: 29–40.

38. **Lagasse E, Connors H, Al-Dhalimy M, et al.** *Purified hematopoietic stem cells can differentiate into hepatocytes in vivo.* Nat Med. 2000; 6: 1229–1234.

39. **Gill M, Dias S, Hattori K, et al.** *Vascular trauma induces rapid but transient mobilization of VEGFR2(+)AC133(+) endothelial precursor cells.* Circ Res. 2001; 88: 167–174.

40. **Etzion S, Battler A, Barbash IM, et al.** *Influence of embryonic cardiomyocyte transplantation on the progression of heart failure in a*

rat model of extensive myocardial infarction. J Mol Cell Cardiol. 2001; 33: 1321–1330.

41. **Guan K, Furst DO, Wobus AM.** *Modulation of sarcomere organization during embryonic stem cell-derived cardiomyocyte differentiation.* Eur J Cell Biol. 1999; 78: 813–823.

42. **Liesveld JL, Rosell K, Panoskaltsis N, et al.** *Response of human CD34+ cells to CXC, CC, and CX3C chemokines: implications for cell migration and activation.* J Hematother Stem Cell Res. 2001; 10: 643–655.

43. **Ying Q-L, Nichols J, Evans E, et al.** *Changing potency by spontaneous fusion.* Nature. 2002; 416: 545–548.

44. **Wagers AJ, Sherwood RI, Christensen JL, et al.** *Little evidence for developmental plasticity of adult hematopoietic stem cells.* Science. 2002; 297: 2256–2259.

45. **Rodney L, Rietze RI, Valcanis H, et al.** *Purification of a pluripotent neural stem cell from the adult mouse brain.* Nature. 2001; 412: 736–739.

46. **Garot J, Unterseeh T, Teiger E, et al.** *Magnetic resonance imaging of targeted catheter-based implantation of myogenic precursor cells into infarcted left ventricular myocardium.* J Am Coll Cardiol. 2003; 41: 1841–1846.

47. **Tse WT, Pendleton JD, Beyer WM, et al.** *Suppression of allogeneic T-cell proliferation by human marrow stromal cells: implications in transplantation.* Transplantation. 2003; 75: 389–397.

48. **Goldstein JA, Demetriou D, Grines CL, et al.** *Multiple complex coronary plaques in patients with acute myocardial infarction.* N Engl J Med. 2000; 343: 915–922.

49. **Rioufol G, Finet G, Ginon I, et al.** *Multiple atherosclerotic plaque rupture in acute coronary syndrome: a three-vessel intravascular ultrasound study.* Circulation. 2002; 106: 804–808.

50. **Forrester JS, Price M, Makkar R.** *Mending the broken heart.* Clin Cardiol. 2003. In press.

51. **Gutierrez-Delgado F, Bensinger W.** *Safety of granulocyte colony-stimulating factor in normal donors.* Curr Opin Hematol. 2001; 8: 155–160.

52. **Zhang YM, Hartzell C, Narlow M, et al.** *Stem cell-derived cardiomyocytes demonstrate arrhythmic potential.* Circulation. 2002; 106: 1294–1299.

53. **Tateishi-Yuyama E, Matsubara H, Murohara T, et al.** *Therapeutic angiogenesis for patients with limb ischemia by autologous transplantation of bone-marrow cells: a pilot study and a ran-*

domised controlled trial. Lancet. 2002; 360: 427–435.

54. **Menasche P, Hagege AA, Scorsin M, et al.** *Myoblast transplantation for heart failure. Lancet.* 2001; 357: 279–280.

55. **Jain M, DerSimonian H, Brenner DA, et al.** *Cell therapy attenuates deleterious ventricular remodeling and improves cardiac performance after myocardial infarction. Circulation.* 2001; 103: 1920–1927.

56. **Rajnoch C, Chachques JC, Berrebi A, et al.** *Cellular therapy reverses myocardial dysfunction.* J Thorac Cardiovasc Surg. 2001; 121: 871–878

57. **Lapidot T, Petit I.** *Current understanding of stem cell mobilization: the roles of chemokines, proteolytic enzymes, adhesion molecules, cytokines, and stromal cells.* Exp Hematol. 2002; 30: 973–981

58. **Jain M, DerSimonian H, Brenner DA, et al.** *Cell therapy attenuates deleterious ventricular remodeling and improves cardiac performance after myocardial infarction. Circulation.* 2001; 103: 1920

59. **Stamm C, Westphal B, Kleine HD, et al.** *Autologous bone-marrow stem-cell transplantation for myocardial regeneration. Lancet.* 2003; 361: 45–46.

60. **Rajnoch C, Chachques JC, Berrebi A, et al.** *Cellular therapy reverses myocardial dysfunction.* J Thorac Cardiovasc Surg. 2001; 121: 87

61. **Bartunek J, Dimmeler S, Drexler H, Fernandez-Aviles F, Galinanes M, Janssens S, Martin J, Mathur A, Menasche P, Priori S, Strauer B, Tendera M, Wijns W, Zeiher A.** *The consensus of the task force of the European Society of Cardiology concerning the clinical investigation of the use of autologous adult stem cells for repair of the heart.* Eur Heart J. 2006 Mar 16; PMID: 16543252

62. Restoration of Cardiac Progenitor Cells After Myocardial Infarction by Self-Proliferation and Selective Homing of Bone Marrow–Derived Stem Cells - **Frédéric Mouquet, Otmar Pfister, Mohit Jain, Angelos Oikonomopoulos, Soeun Ngoy, Ross Summer, Alan Fine, and Ronglih Liao** Circ. Res. 97: 1090 -1092.

63. Bone Marrow Cells Differentiate in Cardiac Cell Lineages After Infarction Independently of Cell Fusion - **Jan Kajstura, Marcello Rota, Brian Whang, Stefano Cascapera, Toru Hosoda, Claudia Bearzi, Daria Nurzynska, Hideko Kasahara, Elias Zias, Massimiliano Bonafé, Bernardo Nadal-Ginard, Daniele Torella, Angelo Nascimbene, Federico Quaini, Konrad Urbanek, Annarosa Leri, and Piero Anversa**Circ. Res. 96: 127 -137;

64. **Shintani S, Murohara T, Ikeda H, et al.** *Mobilization of endothe-*

lial progenitor cells in patients with acute myocardial infarction. Circulation. 2001

65. **Taylor DA, Atkins BZ, Hungspreugs P, et al.** *Regenerating functional myocardium: improved performance after skeletal myoblast transplantation. Nat Med.* 1998; 4: 929–933

66. **Li RK, Welsel RD, Mickle DA, et al.** *Autologous porcine heart cell transplantation improved heart function after a myocardial infarction.* J Thorac Cardiovasc Surg. 2000; 119: 62–68

67. **Penn MS, Francis GS, Ellis SG, et al.** *Autologous cell transplantation for the treatment of damaged myocardium.* Prog Cardiovasc Dis. 2002; 45: 21–32

68. **Yoon Y-A, Murayama T, Tkebuchawa T, et al.** *Clonally expanded bone marrow derived stem cells differentiate into multiple lineages in vitro and can attenuate myocardial dysfunction post myocardial infarction. Circulation.* 2002; 106

69. **Orlic D, Kajstura J, Chimenti S, et al.** *Transplanted adult bone marrow cells repair myocardial infarcts in mice.* Ann NY Acad Sci. 2001; 938: 221–229

70. **Tomita S, Mickle DA, Weisel RD, et al.** *Improved heart function with myogenesis and angiogenesis after autologous porcine bone marrow stromal cell transplantation.* J Thorac Cardiovasc Surg. 2002; 123: 1132–1140

71. **Lapidot T, Petit I.** *Current understanding of stem cell mobilization: the roles of chemokines, proteolytic enzymes, adhesion molecules, cytokines, and stromal cells.* Exp Hematol. 2002; 30: 973–981

72. **Iwaguro H, Yamaguchi J, Kalka C, et al.** *Endothelial progenitor cell vascular endothelial growth factor gene transfer for vascular regeneration. Circulation.* 2002; 105: 732–738.

73. **Shake JG, Gruber PJ, Baumgartner WA, et al.** *Mesenchymal stem cell implantation in a swine myocardial infarct model: engraftment and functional effects.* Ann Thorac Surg. 2002

74. **Reyes M, Dudek A, Jahagirdar B, et al.** *Origin of endothelial progenitors in human postnatal bone marrow.* J Clin Invest. 2002;

75. **Jiang Y, Jahagirdar BN, Reinhardt RL, et al.** *Pluripotency of mesenchymal stem cells derived from adult marrow. Nature.* 2002; 418: 41–49

76. **Devine SM, Bartholomew AM, Mahmud N, et al.** *Mesenchymal stem cells are capable of homing to the bone marrow of non-human primates following systemic infusion.* Exp Hematol. 2001; 29: 244–

77. **Rioufol G, Finet G, Ginon I, et al.** *Multiple atherosclerotic plaque rupture in acute coronary syndrome: a three-vessel intravascular*

ultrasound study. Circulation. 2002; 106: 804–808

78. **Forrester JS, Price M, Makkar R.** *Mending the broken heart. Clin Cardiol.* 2003

79. **Menasche P, Hagege AA, Scorsin M, et al.** *Myoblast transplantation for heart failure. Lancet.* 2001; 357: 279–280

80. **Stamm C, Westphal B, Kleine HD, et al.** *Autologous bone-marrow stem-cell transplantation for myocardial regeneration. Lancet.* 2003

81. **Assmus B, Schachinger V, Teupe C, et al.** *Transplantation of Progenitor Cells and Regeneration Enhancement in Acute Myocardial Infarction (TOPCARE-AMI). Circulation.* 2002; 106: 3009–3017

82. **Fuchs S, Weisz G, Kornowski R, et al.** *Catheter-based autologous bone marrow myocardial injection in no-option patients with advanced coronary artery disease: a feasibility and safety study. Circulation.* 2002; 106 (suppl II): II-655–II-656.

83. **Jain M, DerSimonian H, Brenner DA, et al.** *Cell therapy attenuates deleterious ventricular remodeling and improves cardiac performance after myocardial infarction. Circulation.* 2001; 103: 1920–

84. **Rajnoch C, Chachques JC, Berrebi A, et al.** *Cellular therapy reverses myocardial dysfunction. J Thorac Cardiovasc Surg.* 2001; 121: 871–878

85. **Jiang Y, Jahagirdar BN, Reinhardt RL, et al.** *Pluripotency of mesenchymal stem cells derived from adult marrow. Nature.* 2002; 418 85

86. **Fuchs S, Weisz G, Kornowski R, et al.** *Catheter-based autologous bone marrow myocardial injection in no-option patients with advanced coronary artery disease: a feasibility and safety study. Circulation.* 2002; 106

Mesenchymal Stem Cells

1. **Shake JG, Gruber PJ, Baumgartner WA, et al.** *Mesenchymal stem cell implantation in a swine myocardial infarct model: engraftment and functional effects.* Ann Thorac Surg. 2002

2. **Shake JG, Gruber PJ, Baumgartner WA, et al.** *Mesenchymal stem cell implantation in a swine myocardial infarct model: engraftment and functional effects.* Ann Thorac Surg. 2002; 73: 1919–1925

3. **Jiang Y, Jahagirdar BN, Reinhardt RL, et al.** *Pluripotency of mesenchymal stem cells derived from adult marrow. Nature.* 2002; 418: 41–49

4. **Devine SM, Bartholomew AM, Mahmud N, et al.** *Mesenchymal stem cells are capable of homing to the bone marrow of non-human primates following systemic infusion.* Exp Hematol.

2001; 29: 244–255
5. **Shake JG, Gruber PJ, Baumgartner WA, et al.** *Mesenchymal stem cell implantation in a swine myocardial infarct model: engraftment and functional effects.* Ann Thorac Surg. 2002; 73: 1919–1925.
6. **Jager M, Bachmann R, Scharfstadt A, Krauspe R.** *Ovine cord blood accommodates multipotent mesenchymal progenitor cells.* In Vivo. 2006 Mar-Apr;20(2):205-14. PMID: 16634520

Progenitor

1. **Frédéric Mouquet, Otmar Pfister, Mohit Jain, Angelos Oikonomopoulos, Soeun Ngoy, Ross Summer, Alan Fine, and Ronglih Liao.** *Restoration of Cardiac Progenitor Cells After Myocardial Infarction by Self-Proliferation and Selective Homing of Bone Marrow–Derived Stem Cells.* Circ. Res. 97: 1090 -1092; published online before print as doi:10.1161/01.RES.0000194330.66545.f5
2. **Frédéric Mouquet, Otmar Pfister, Mohit Jain, Angelos Oikonomopoulos, Soeun Ngoy, Ross Summer, Alan Fine, and Ronglih Liao.** *Restoration of Cardiac Progenitor Cells After Myocardial Infarction by Self-Proliferation and Selective Homing of Bone Marrow-Derived Stem Cells.* Circ. Res. published November 3, 2005, doi: 10.1161/01.RES.0000194330.66545
3. **Shintani S, Murohara T, Ikeda H, et al.** *Mobilization of endothelial progenitor cells in patients with acute myocardial infarction.* Circulation. 2001
4. **Iwaguro H, Yamaguchi J, Kalka C, et al.** *Endothelial progenitor cell vascular endothelial growth factor gene transfer for vascular regeneration.* Circulation. 2002; 105: 732–738.
5. **Reyes M, Dudek A, Jahagirdar B, et al.** *Origin of endothelial progenitors in human postnatal bone marrow.* J Clin Invest. 2002;
6. **Assmus B, Schachinger V, Teupe C, et al.** *Transplantation of progenitor cells and regeneration enhancement in acute myocardial infarction. Transplantation of Progenitor Cells and Regeneration Enhancement in Acute Myocardial Infarction (TOPCARE-AMI).* Circulation. 2002; 106: 3009–3017
7. **Yasuhara T, Matsukawa N, Yu G, Xu L, Mays RW, Kovach J, Deans RJ, Hess DC, Carroll JE, Borlongan CV.** *Behavioral and histological characterization of intrahippocampal grafts of human bone marrow-derived multipotent progenitor cells in neonatal rats with hypoxic-ischemic injury.* Cell Transplant. 2006;15(3):231-8.
8. **Galli D, Innocenzi A, Staszewsky L, Zanetta L, Sampaolesi M,**

Bai A, Martinoli E, Carlo E, Balconi G, Fiordaliso F, Chimenti S, Cusella G, Dejana E, Cossu G, Latini R. *Mesoangioblasts, vessel-associated multipotent stem cells, repair the infarcted heart by multiple cellular mechanisms: a comparison with bone marrow progenitors, fibroblasts, and endothelial cells.*

9. **Shintani S, Murohara T, Ikeda H, et al.** *Mobilization of endothelial progenitor cells in patients with acute myocardial infarction.* Circulation. 2001; 103: 2776–2779.

10. **Heissig B, Hattori K, Dias S, et al.** *Recruitment of stem and progenitor cells from the bone marrow niche requires MMP-9 mediated release of kit-ligand.*

11. **Iwaguro H, Yamaguchi J, Kalka C, et al.** *Endothelial progenitor cell vascular endothelial growth factor gene transfer for vascular regeneration. Circulation.* 2002; 105: 732–

12. **Assmus B, Schachinger V, Teupe C, et al.** *Transplantation of Progenitor Cells and Regeneration Enhancement in Acute Myocardial Infarction (TOPCARE-AMI).*

13. **Shintani S, Murohara T, Ikeda H, et al.** *Mobilization of endothelial progenitor cells in patients with acute myocardial infarction.* Circulation. 2001; 103: 2776–2779.

14. **Heissig B, Hattori K, Dias S, et al.** *Recruitment of stem and progenitor cells from the bone marrow niche requires MMP-9 mediated release of kit-ligand.* Cell. 2002; 109: 625–637.

Adult Stem Cells

1. **Graf T.** *Differentiation plasticity of hematopoietic cells.* Blood. 2002; 99: 3089–3101.

2. **Malouf NN, Coleman WB, Girsham JW, et al.** *Adult-derived stem cells from the liver become myocytes in the heart in vivo.* Am J Pathol. 2001; 158: 1929–1935.

3. **Donovan PJ, Gearhart J.** *The end of the beginning for pluripotent stem cells. Nature.* 2001; 414: 92–97.

4. **Jackson KA, Majka SM, Wulf GG, et al.** *Stem cells: a mini review.* J Cell Biochem. 2002; (suppl 38): 1–6.

5. **Orlic D, Hill JM, Arai AE.** *Stem cells for myocardial regeneration.* Circ Res. 2002; 91: 1092–1102.

6. **Bartunek J, Dimmeler S, Drexler H, Fernandez-Aviles F, Galinanes M, Janssens S, Martin J, Mathur A, Menasche P, Priori S, Strauer B, Tendera M, Wijns W, Zeiher A.** *The consensus of the task force of the European Society of Cardiology concern-*

ing the clinical investigation of the use of autologous adult stem cells for repair of the heart. Eur Heart J. 2006 Mar 16; [Epub ahead of print]. PMID: 16543252 [PubMed - as supplied by publisher]

7. **D'Ambrosio A, did Sciascio G.** *Transcatheter cell therapy of heart failure: state of the art.* G Ital Cardiol (Rome). 2006 Jan;7(1):23-39. Italian PMID: 16528960 [PubMed - in process]

8. **Sheikh AY, Wu JC.** *Molecular imaging of cardiac stem cell transplantation.* Curr Cardiol Rep. 2006 Mar;8(2):147-54. PMID: 16524542 [PubMed - in process]

9. **Aceves JL, Archundia A, Diaz G, Paez A, Masso F, Alvarado M, Lopez M, Aceves R, Ixcamparij C, Puente A, Vilchis R, Montano LF.** *Stem cell perspectives in myocardial infarctions.* Rev Invest Clin. 2005 Mar-Apr;57(2):156-62. Spanish. PMID: 16524054 [PubMed - in process]

10. **Zhang N, Mustin D, Reardon W, Almeida AD, Mozdziak P, Mrug M, Eisenberg LM, Sedmera D.** *Blood-borne stem cells differentiate into vascular and cardiac lineages during normal development.* Stem Cells Dev. 2006 Feb;15(1):17-28. PMID: 16522159 [PubMed - in process]

11. **Van Haaften T, Thebaud B.** *Adult Bone Marrow-Derived Stem Cells for the Lung: Implications for Pediatric Lung Diseases.* Pediatr Res. 2006 Mar 2; [Epub ahead of print] PMID: 16514220 [PubMed - as supplied by publisher]

12. **Schulze M, Fandrich F, Ungefroren H, Kremer B.** *Adult stem cells—perspectives in treatment of metabolic diseases.* Acta Gastroenterol Belg. 2005 Oct-Dec;68(4):461-5. PMID: 16433004

13. **Yen BL, Huang HI, Chien CC, Jui HY, Ko BS, Yao M, Shun CT, Yen ML, Lee MC, Chen YC.** *Isolation of multipotent cells from human term placenta.* Stem Cells. 2005;23(1):3-9. PMID: 15625118

14. **Rice CM, Scolding NJ.** *Adult stem cells—reprogramming neurological repair?* Lancet. 2004 Jul 10-16;364(9429):193-9. Review. PMID: 15246733

15. **Principal Investigator: Raj Makkar, MD Co-Investigators: P.K. Shah, MD; Stephen Lim, MD; Michael Lee, MD; Michael Lill, MD.** *Randomized Evaluation of Intracoronary Transplantation of Bone Marrow Stem Cells in Myocardial Infarction (Revitalize) Trial*

16. **Bartunek J, Dimmeler S, Drexler H, Fernandez-Aviles F, Galinanes M, Janssens S, Martin J, Mathur A, Menasche P, Priori S, Strauer B, Tendera M, Wijns W, Zeiher A.** *The consensus of the task force of the European Society of Cardiology concerning the clinical investigation of the use of autologous adult stem cells*

for repair of the heart.
Eur Heart J. 2006 Mar 16; PMID: 16543252

17. **Jan Kajstura, Marcello Rota, Brian Whang, Stefano Cascapera, Toru Hosoda, Claudia Bearzi, Daria Nurzynska, Hideko Kasahara, Elias Zias, Massimiliano Bonafé, Bernardo Nadal-Ginard, Daniele Torella, Angelo Nascimbene, Federico Quaini, Konrad Urbanek, Annarosa Leri, and Piero Anversa.** *Bone Marrow Cells Differentiate in Cardiac Cell Lineages After Infarction Independently of Cell Fusion.* Circ. Res. 96: 127 -137;

18. **Orlic D, Hill JM, Arai AE.** *Stem cells for myocardial regeneration.* Circ Res. 2002; 91: 1092

Bone Marrow Stem Cells

1. **Jan Kajstura, Marcello Rota, Brian Whang, Stefano Cascapera, Toru Hosoda, Claudia Bearzi, Daria Nurzynska, Hideko Kasahara, Elias Zias, Massimiliano Bonafé, Bernardo Nadal-Ginard, Daniele Torella, Angelo Nascimbene, Federico Quaini, Konrad Urbanek, Annarosa Leri, and Piero Anversa.** *Bone Marrow Cells Differentiate in Cardiac Cell Lineages After Infarction Independently of Cell Fusion.* Circ. Res. 96: 127 -137; published online before print as doi:10.1161/01.RES.0000151843.79801.60

2. **Trial Principal Investigator: Raj Makkar, MD, Co-Investigators: P.K. Shah, MD; Stephen Lim, MD; Michael Lee, MD; Michael Lill, MD.** *Randomized Evaluation of Intracoronary Transplantation of Bone Marrow Stem Cells in Myocardial Infarction (Revitalize)*

3. **Yoon Y-A, Murayama T, Tkebuchawa T, et al.** *Clonally expanded bone marrow derived stem cells differentiate into multiple lineages in vitro and can attenuate myocardial dysfunction post myocardial infarction. Circulation.* 2002; 106 (suppl II): II–51.

4. **Lewis E, Qu X, Nakao M, et al.** *transdifferentiation. Circulation.* 2001; 104 (suppl II): II–2829.

5. **Fuchs S, Baffour R, Zhou YF, et al.** *Transendocardial delivery of autologous bone marrow enhances collateral perfusion and regional function in pigs with chronic experimental myocardial ischemia.* J Am Coll Cardiol. 2001; 37: 1726–1732.

6. **Orlic D, Kajstura J, Chimenti S, et al.** *Transplanted adult bone marrow cells repair myocardial infarcts in mice.* Ann NY Acad Sci. 2001; 938: 221–229

7. **Wang JS, Shum-Tim D, Chedrawy E, et al.** *The coronary delivery of marrow stromal cells for myocardial regeneration: pathophysio-*

logic and therapeutic implications. J Thorac Cardiovasc Surg. 2001; 122: 699–705

8. **Tomita S, Mickle DA, Weisel RD, et al.** *Improved heart function with myogenesis and angiogenesis after autologous porcine bone marrow stromal cell transplantation.* J Thorac Cardiovasc Surg. 2002; 123: 1132–1140

9. **Orlic D, Kajstura J, Chimenti S, et al.** *Mobilized bone marrow cells repair the infarcted heart, improving function and survival.* Proc Natl Acad Sci U S A. 2001; 98: 10344–10349.

10. **Wagers AJ, Sherwood RI, Christensen JL, et al.** *Little evidence for developmental plasticity of adult hematopoietic stem cells.* Science. 2002; 297: 2256–2259.

11. **Terada N, Hamazaki T, Oka M, et al.** *Bone marrow cells adopt phenotype of other cells by spontaneous cell fusion.* Nature. 2002; 416: 542–545.

12. **Tomoda H, Aoki N.** *Bone marrow stimulation and left ventricular function in acute myocardial infarction.* Clin Cardiol. 2003. In press.

13. **Stamm C, Westphal B, Kleine HD, et al.** *Autologous bone-marrow stem-cell transplantation for myocardial regeneration.* Lancet. 2003; 361: 45–46.

14. **Hamano K, Nishida M, Hirata K.** *Local implantation of autologous bone marrow cells for therapeutic angiogenesis in patients with ischemic heart disease: clinical trial and preliminary results.* Jpn Circ J. 2001; 65: 845–847.

15. **Strauer BE, Brehm M, Zeus T, et al.** *Repair of infarcted myocardium by autologus intracoronary mononuclear bone marrow cell transplantation in humans.* Circulation. 2002; 106: 1913–1918.

16. **Fuchs S, Weisz G, Kornowski R, et al.** *Catheter-based autologous bone marrow myocardial injection in no-option patients with advanced coronary artery disease: a feasibility and safety study.* Circulation. 2002; 106 (suppl II): II-655–II-656.

17. **Yoon Y-A, Murayama T, Tkebuchawa T, et al.** *Clonally expanded bone marrow derived stem cells differentiate into multiple lineages in vitro and can attenuate myocardial dysfunction post myocardial infarction.* Circulation. 2002; 106 (suppl II): II–51.

18. **Lewis E, Qu X, Nakao M, et al.** *Cardiac differentiation markers do not support the ability of bone marrow cells to undergo in vitro transdifferentiation.* Circulation. 2001; 104 (suppl II): II–2829.

19. **Fuchs S, Baffour R, Zhou YF, et al.** *Transendocardial delivery of autologous bone marrow enhances collateral perfusion and regional function in pigs with chronic experimental myocardial ischemia.* J

Am Coll Cardiol. 2001; 37: 1726–1732.

20. **Orlic D, Kajstura J, Chimenti S, et al.** *Transplanted adult bone marrow cells repair myocardial infarcts in mice.* Ann NY Acad Sci. 2001; 938: 221–229

21. **Wang JS, Shum-Tim D, Chedrawy E, et al.** *The coronary delivery of marrow stromal cells for myocardial regeneration: pathophysiologic and therapeutic implications.* J Thorac Cardiovasc Surg. 2001; 122: 699–705

22. **Tomita S, Mickle DA, Weisel RD, et al.** *Improved heart function with myogenesis and angiogenesis after autologous porcine bone marrow stromal cell transplantation.* J Thorac Cardiovasc Surg. 2002; 123: 1132–1140

23. **Kocher AA, Schuster MD, Szaboles MJ, et al.** *Neovascularization of ischemic myocardium by human bone-marrow-derived angioblasts prevents cardiomyocyte apoptosis, reduces remodeling and improves cardiac function.* Nat Med. 2001; 7: 430–436.

24. **Orlic D, Kajstura J, Chimentl S, et al.** *Mobilized bone marrow cells repair the infarcted heart, improving function and survival.* Proc Natl Acad Sci U S A. 2001; 98: 10344–10349.

25. **Tomoda H, Aokl N.** *Bone marrow stimulation and left ventricular function in acute myocardial infarction.* Clin Cardiol. 2003. In press.

26. **Terada N, Hamazaki T, Oka M, et al.** *Bone marrow cells adopt phenotype of other cells by spontaneous cell fusion. Nature.* 2002; 416: 542–545.

27. **Yoon Y-A, Murayama T, Tkebuchawa T, et al.** *Clonally expanded bone marrow derived stem cells differentiate into multiple lineages in vitro and can attenuate myocardial dysfunction post myocardial infarction. Circulation.* 2002; 106

28. **Orlic D, Kajstura J, Chimenti S, et al.** *Transplanted adult bone marrow cells repair myocardial infarcts in mice.* Ann NY Acad Sci. 2001; 938: 221–229

29. **Tomita S, Mickle DA, Weisel RD, et al.** *Improved heart function with myogenesis and angiogenesis after autologous porcine bone marrow stromal cell transplantation.*

Diabetes

1. **Klibansky DA, Chin A, Duignan IJ, Edelberg JM.** *Synergistic targeting with bone marrow-derived cells and PDGF improves diabetic vascular function.* Am J Physiol Heart Circ Physiol. 2006 Apr;290(4):H1387-92. Epub 2005 Dec 9. PMID: 16339836 [PubMed - in process]

2. **Sassa M, Fukuda K, Fujimoto S, Toyoda K, Fujita Y, Matsumoto S, Okitsu T, Iwanaga Y, Noguchi H, Nagata H, Yonekawa Y, Ohara T, Okamoto M, Tanaka K, Seino Y, Inagaki N, Yamada Y.** *A single transplantation of the islets can produce glycemic stability and reduction of basal insulin requirement.* Diabetes Res Clin Pract. 2006 Apr 4; [Epub ahead of print] PMID: 16600414 [PubMed - as supplied by publisher]

3. **Somjen D, Shen M, Stern N, Mirsky N.** *Diabetes modulates differentially creatine kinase-specific activity responsiveness to estradiol-17beta and to raloxifene in rat organs.* J Cell Biochem. 2006 Apr 5; [Epub ahead of print]. PMID: 16598752 [PubMed - as supplied by publisher]

4. **Leschke M, Schwenk B, Bollinger C, Faehling M.** *Impaired glucose metabolism in patients with ischaemic heart disease.* Clin Res Cardiol. 2006 Jan;95 Suppl 1:i98-i102. German. PMID: 16598558 [PubMed - in process]

5. **Diehm C, Lawall H.** *Diabetes, heart surgery and the peripheral arteries.* Clin Res Cardiol. 2006 Jan;95(Supplement 1):i63-i69. German. PMID: 16598551 [PubMed - as supplied by publisher]

6. **Fetter M.** *Diabetes and cerebrovascular disease.* Clin Res Cardiol. 2006 Jan;95 Suppl 1:i59-i62. German. PMID: 16598550 [PubMed - in process]

7. **Loebe M, Ramasubbu K, Hamilton DJ.** *Diabetes and heart transplantation.* Clin Res Cardiol. 2006 Jan;95 Suppl 1:i48-i53. German. PMID: 16598548 [PubMed - in process]

8. **Arnrich B, Albert A, Walter J.** Risk stratification of patients with diabetes mellitus *undergoing coronary artery bypass grafting-a comparison of statistical methods.* Clin Res Cardiol. 2006 Jan;95 Suppl 1:i14-i17. German. PMID: 16598542 [PubMed - in process]

9. **Jacob S, Lauruschkat AH, Lippmann-Grob B.** *Heart-Diabetes-Network-A concept for improved care for diabetic cardiovascular patients following cardiac surgical intervention.* Clin Res Cardiol. 2006 Jan;95 Suppl 1:i125-i129. German. PMID: 16598539 [PubMed - in process]

10. **Miche E, Herrmann G, Nowak M, Wirtz U, Tietz M, Hurst M, Zoller B, Radzewitz A.** *Effect of an exercise training program on endothelial dysfunction in diabetic and non-diabetic patients with severe chronic heart failure.* Clin Res Cardiol. 2006 Jan;95(Supplement 1):i117-i124. Diabetologia. 2006 Apr 4; [Epub ahead of print] PMID: 16586069 [PubMed - as supplied by publisher]

11. **Itoh S, Ding B, Shishido T, Lerner-Marmarosh N, Wang N, Maekawa N, Berk BC, Takeishi Y, Yan C, Blaxall BC, Abe JI.** *Role of p90 Ribosomal S6 Kinase-Mediated Prorenin-Converting Enzyme in Ischemic and Diabetic Myocardium.Circulation.* 2006 Apr 3; [Epub ahead of print] PMID: 16585392 [PubMed - as supplied by publisher]

12. **Wan Q, Harris MF, Jayasinghe UW, Flack J, Georgiou A, Penn DL, Burns JR.** *Quality of diabetes care and coronary heart disease absolute risk in patients with type II diabetes mellitus in Australian general practice.* Qual Saf Health Care. 2006 Apr;15(2):131-5. PMID: 16585115 [PubMed - in process]

13. **Costa J, Borges M, David C, Carneiro AV.** *Efficacy of lipid lowering drug treatment for diabetic and non-diabetic patients: meta-analysis of randomised controlled trials.BMJ.* 2006 Apr 3; [Epub ahead of print]

Policosonal

1. **Menendez R, Amor AM, Rodeiro I, et al.** *Policosanol modulates HMG-CoA reductase activity in cultured fibroblasts.* Arch Med Res 2001 Jan-Feb;32(1):8-12.

2. **Menendez R, Amor AM, Gonzalez RM, Fraga V, Mas R.** *Effect of policosanol on the hepatic cholesterol biosynthesis of normocholesterolemic rats.* Biol Res 1996;29(2):253-7

3. **Menendez R, Fernandez SI, Del Rio A, et al.** *Policosanol inhibits cholesterol biosynthesis and enhances low density lipoprotein processing in cultured human fibroblasts.* Biol Res 1994

4. **Janikula M.**Policosanol: a new treatment for cardiovascular disease? Altern Med Rev 2002 Jun;7(3):203-17

5. **Arruzazabala ML, Noa M, Menendez R, et al.** *Protective effect of policosanol on atherosclerotic lesions in rabbits with exogenous hypercholesterolemia.* Braz J Med Biol Res 2000 Jul;33(7):835-40

6. **Mirkin A, Mas R, Martinto M, Boccanera R, Robertis A, Poudes R, Fuster A, Lastreto E, Yanez M, Irico G, McCook B, Farre A.** *Efficacy and tolerability of policosanol in hypercholesterolemic postmenopausal women.* Int J Clin Pharmacol Res 2001;21(1):31-41.

7. **Janikula M.** *Policosanol: a new treatment for cardiovascular disease?* Altern Med Rev 2002 Jun;7(3):203-17.

8. **Gouni-Berthold I, Berthold HK.** *Policosanol: clinical pharmacology and therapeutic significance of a new lipid-lowering agent.* Am Heart J 2002 Feb;143(2):356-65.

Low Cholesterol and Violent, Hostile, Aggressive Behavior and Suicide

1. **Zhang J, et al.** *Association of Serum Cholesterol and History of School Suspension among School-age Children and Adolescents in the United States.* American Journal of Epidemiology, Apr 1, 2005; 161 (7): 691-699.
2. **Markovitz JH, et al.** *Lack of relations of hostility, negative affect, and high-risk behavior with low plasma lipid levels in the Coronary Artery Risk Development in Young Adults Study.* Archives of Internal Medicine, 1997; 157: 1953-1959.
3. **Repo-Tiihomen E, et al.** *Total serum cholesterol level, violent criminal offences, suicidal behavior, mortality and the appearance of conduct disorder in Finnish male criminal offenders with antisocial personality disorder.* European Archives Of Psychiatry And Clinical Neuroscience, 2002; 252: 8-11.
4. **Vevera J, et al.** *Cholesterol concentrations in violent and non-violent women suicide attempters.* European Psychiatry, 2003; 18: 23-7.
5. **Golomb BA, et al.** *Low cholesterol and violent crime.* Journal of Psychiatric Research, 2000; 34: 301-309.
6. **Hillbrand M, et al.** *Serum cholesterol and aggression in hospitalized male forensic patients.* Journal of Behavioral Medicine, 1995; 18: 33-43.
7. **Hillbrand M, et al.** *Serum cholesterol concentrations and mood states in violent psychiatric patients: an experience sampling study.* Journal of Behavioral Medicine, 2000; 23: 519-529.
8. **Mufti RM, et al.** *Low cholesterol and violence.* Psychiatric Services, 1998; 49: 221-224.
9. **Kaplan JR, et al.** *The effects of fat and cholesterol on social behavior in monkeys.* Psychosomatic Medicine, 1991; 53: 634-642.

C-Reactive Protein (CRP)

1. **Pepys MG.** *The acute phase response and C-reactive protein.: Weatherall DJ, Ledingham JGG, Warrell DA, eds. Oxford Textbook of Medicine.* 3rd ed. Oxford, England: Oxford University Press; 1995:1527–1533.
2. **Ridker PM, Rifai N, Pfeffer M, et al.** *Long-term effects of pravastatin on plasma concentration of C-reactive protein. Circulation.* 1999;100:230–235
3. **Ewart HKM, Ridker PM, Rifai N, et al.** *Absence of diurnal varia-*

tion of C-reactive protein levels in healthy human subjects. Clin Chem. 2001;47:426–430

4. **Ridker PM, Hennekens CH, Rifai N, et al.** *Hormone replacement therapy and increased plasma concentration of C-reactive protein. Circulation. 1999;100:713–716.*

5. **Cushman M, Legault C, Barrett-Connor E, et al.** *Effect of post-menopausal hormones on inflammation sensitive proteins: the Postmenopausal Estrogen/Progestin Interventions (PEPI) Study. Circulation. 1999;100:717–722.*

6. **Van Baal WM, Kenemans P, van der Mooren MJ, et al.** *Increased C-reactive protein levels during short-term hormone replacement therapy in healthy postmenopausal women.* Thromb Haemost. 1998;81:925–928.

7. **Visser M, Bouter LM, McQuillen GM, et al.** Elevated C-reactive protein levels in overweight and obese adults. J AMA. 1999;282:2131–2135.

8. **Yudkin JS, Stehouwer CDA, Emeis JJ, et al.** *C-reactive protein in healthy subjects: associations with obesity, insulin resistance, and endothelial dysfunction: a potential role for cytokines originating from adipose tissue?* Arterioscler Thromb Vasc Biol. 1999;19:972–978

9. **Ridker PM, Rifai N, Stampfer MJ, et al.** *Plasma concentration of interleukin-6 and the risk of future myocardial infarction among apparently healthy men. Circulation. 2000;101:1767–1772.*

10. **Ridker PM, Rifai N, Pfeffer M, et al, for the Cholesterol And Recurrent Events (CARE) Investigators.** *Elevation of tumor necrosis factor-alpha and increased risk of recurrent coronary events after myocardial infarction. Circulation. 2000;101:2149–2153*

11. **Smith JK, Dykes R, Douglas JE, et al.** *Long-term exercise and atherogenic activity of blood mononuclear cells in persons at risk of developing ischemic heart disease.* JAMA. 1999;281:1722–1727.

12. **Ford CS.** *Body mass index, diabetes, and C-reactive protein among U.S. adults.* Diabetes Care. 1999;22:1971–

13. **Festa A, D'Agostino R, Howard G, et al.** *Chronic subclinical inflammation as part of the insulin resistance syndrome: the Insulin Resistance Atherosclerosis Study (IRAS). Circulation. 2000;102:42–47.*

14. **Sesmilo G, Biller BMK, Llevadot J, et al.** *Effects of growth hormone administration on inflammatory and other cardiovascular risk markers in men with growth hormone deficiency.* Ann Intern Med. 2000;133:111–122.

15. **Downs JR, Clearfield M, Weis S, et al, for the AFCAPS/TexCAPS Research Group.** *Primary prevention of acute coronary events with lovastatin in men and women with average cholesterol levels: results of AFCAPS/TexCAPS.* JAMA. 1998;279:1615–1622. .

16. **Pasceri V, Willerson JT, Yeh ET.** *Direct proinflammatory effect of C-reactive protein on human endothelial cells. Circulation.* 2000;102:2165–2168.

17. **Ridker PM, Rifai N, Rose L, Buring JE, Cook NR.** *Comparison of C-reactive protein and low-density lipoprotein cholesterol levels in the prediction of first cardiovascular events.* N Engl J Med. 2002;347:1557-1565.

18. **Koenig W, Lowel H, Baumert J, Meisinger C.** *C-reactive protein modulates risk prediction based on the Framingham score: implications for future risk assessment: results from a large cohort study in southern Germany. Circulation.* 2004;109:1349-

19. **Ridker PM, Rifai N, Cook NR, Bradwin G, Buring JE.** *Non-HDL cholesterol, apolipoproteins A-I and B100, standard lipid measures, lipid ratios, and CRP as risk factors for cardiovascular disease in women.* JAMA. 2005;294:326-333.

20. **Pradhan AD, Manson JE, Rifai N, Buring JE, Ridker PM.** *C-reactive protein, interleukin 6, and risk of developing type II diabetes mellitus.* JAMA. 2001;286:327-334.

21. **Ridker PM, Buring JE, Cook NR, Rifai N.** *C-reactive protein, the metabolic syndrome, and risk of incident cardiovascular events: an 8-year follow-up of 14,719 initially healthy American women. Circulation* 2003;107:391-397.

22. **Sesso HD, Buring JE, Rifai N, Blake GJ, Gaziano JM, Ridker PM.** *C-reactive protein and the risk of developing hypertension.* JAMA. 2003;290:2945-2951.

23. **Ridker PM, Rifai N, Pfeffer MA, Sacks F, Braunwald E.** *Long-term effects of pravastatin on plasma concentration of C-reactive protein. Circulation.* 1999;100:230-235.

24. **Ridker PM, Rifai N, Pfeffer MA, et al.** *Inflammation, pravastatin, and the risk of coronary events after myocardial infarction in patients with average cholesterol levels. Circulation.* 1998;98:839-844.

25. **Ridker PM, Rifai N, Clearfield M, et al.** *Measurement of C-reactive protein for the targeting of statin therapy in the primary prevention of acute coronary events.* N Engl J Med. 2001;344:1959-1965.

26. **Ridker PM, Cannon CP, Morrow D, et al.** *C-reactive protein levels and outcomes after statin therapy.* N Engl J Med. 2005;352:20-28.

27. **Nissen SE, Tuzcu EM, Schoenhagen P, et al.** *Statin therapy, LDL cholesterol, C-reactive protein, and coronary artery disease.* N Engl J Med. 2005;352:29-38.

28. **Pearson TA, Mensah GA, Alexander RW.** *Markers of inflammation and cardiovascular disease: application to clinical and public health practice: a statement for healthcare professionals from the Centers for Disease Control and Prevention and the American Heart Association. Circulation.* 2003;107:499-511

Vulnerable Plaque

1. From Vulnerable Plaque to Vulnerable Patient-Part III: Executive Summary of the Screening for Heart Attack Prevention and Education (SHAPE) Task Force Report.Am J Cardiol. 2006 Jul 17;98(2 Suppl 1):2-15. Epub 2006 Jun 12. **Naghavi M, Falk E, Hecht HS, Jamieson MJ, Kaul S, Berman D, Fayad Z, Budoff MJ, Rumberger J, Naqvi TZ, Shaw LJ, Faergeman O, Cohn J, Bahr R, Koenig W, Demirovic J, Arking D, Herrera VL, Badimon J, Goldstein JA, Rudy Y, Airaksinen J, Schwartz RS, Riley WA, Mendes RA, Douglas P, Shah PK; for the SHAPE Task Force.** PMID: 16843744

2. From the single vulnerable plaque, to the multiple complex coronary plaques. From their basis, to the modern therapeutic approach. A clinical reality in the spectrum of the acute coronary syndromes]Arch Cardiol Mex. 2006 Jan-Mar;76 Suppl 1:S6-34. **Lupi Herrera E, Chuquiure Valenzuela E, Gaspar J, Ferez Santander SM.**

3. Sources of error and interpretation of plaque morphology by optical coherence tomography.Am J Cardiol. 2006 Jul 15;98(2):156-9. Epub 2006 May 19. PMID: 16828584 **Manfrini O, Mont E, Leone O, Arbustini E, Eusebi V, Virmani R, Bugiardini R.**

4. C-reactive protein in vulnerable coronary plaques.J Clin Pathol. 2006 Jun 21; [Epub ahead of print] PMID: 16790690 **Norja S, Nuutila L, Karhunen PJ, Goebeler S.**

5. Number of yellow plaques detected in a coronary artery is associated with future risk of acute coronary syndrome: detection of vulnerable patients by angioscopy. J Am Coll Cardiol. 2006 Jun 6;47(11):2194-200. Epub 2006 May 15. PMID: 16750684 **Ohtani T, Ueda Y, Mizote I, Oyabu J, Okada K, Hirayama A, Kodama K.**

6. Intravascular ultrasound-based imaging of vasa vasorum for the detection of vulnerable atherosclerotic plaque. Med Image Comput Comput Assist Interv Int Conf Med Image Comput Comput Assist Interv. 2005;8(Pt 1):343-51. PMID: 16685864 **O'Malley SM, Vavuranakis M, Naghavi M, Kakadiaris IA.**

7. Ruptured vulnerable coronary plaque and Tc-99m sestamibi-based assessment of infarct size.Clin Nucl Med. 2006 Jun;31(6):331-2. PMID: 16714891 **=Wessely R, Bradaric C, Seybold S.**